Suzi

Good night, sweetheart,

Carl

Dec 25, 1974

Insomniacs of the World
Goodnight

Illustrations by Michael K. Frith

 RANDOM HOUSE / NEW YORK

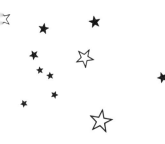

Insomniacs of the World
Goodnight

A BEDSIDE BOOK

Written and Edited
by HILARY RUBINSTEIN

Library of Congress Cataloging in Publication Data

Rubinstein, Hilary.
  Insomniacs of the world, goodnight.

  1. Insomnia. 2. Sleep. I. Title.
RC548.R8   616.8′49   74–9079
ISBN 0–394–48998–5

Manufactured in the United States of America
9 8 7 6 5 4 3 2
First Edition

For HELGE

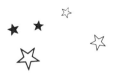

Acknowledgments

In the writing and editing of this book, I have been assisted by many more individuals than I can hope to thank by name here. Many hundreds of people wrote to tell me of their insomniac experiences and remedies, often at length, and I should like to offer a corporate apology now for having replied to most of these letters with little more than a brief acknowledgment; to have answered in kind would on occasions have been a full-time occupation. And I am naturally very grateful to all who have contributed to the chapter on "Ways of Wooing Sleep."

I am particularly indebted to Dr. Christopher Evans for allowing me to reprint "The Function of Dreaming," which was originally published in *Transaction*, to Nancy Phelan for writing specially for this book the chapter on "Yoga and the Art of Relaxation" and to Dr. R. T. Wilkinson for reading the chapter on "How We Sleep and Why We Sleep." Among others whose suggestions and comments were particularly helpful, I would mention: Heather Bradley, Professor Dugal Campbell, Roy Fuller, Jack Goodman, Maureen Kilroe, Albert

Lowy, Herb Mitgang, Hugh Mullins, Patsy Ratner and Paul Vaughan.

For permission to use copyright material, I am grateful to the following: Yale University Press for extracts from *The Function of Sleep*, by Ernest L. Hartmann (copyright © 1973 by Yale University); Bill Berger Associates, Inc., and Longman Group Ltd. for the chapter on "Electrosleep" and "A Sleep Questionnaire," both from *Insomnia*, by Gay Gaer Luce and Julius Segal (copyright © 1968, 1969 by Gay Gaer Luce and Julius Segal); Random House, Inc., Chatto & Windus Ltd. and Mr. George Scott-Moncrieff for the extract from *Swann's Way*, reprinted from *Remembrance of Things Past*, by Marcel Proust, translated by C. K. Scott-Moncrieff (copyright 1934 and renewed © 1962 by Random House, Inc.); Schocken Books, Inc., and Martin Secker & Warburg Ltd. for the extract from *The Diaries of Franz Kafka 1910–1913*, edited by Max Brod, translated by Joseph Kresh (copyright 1948 by Schocken Books, Inc.); A. D. Peters & Co. for the extract from *The Ordeal of Gilbert Pinfold*, by Evelyn Waugh, originally published by Chapman & Hall Ltd., London; Hawthorn Books, Inc., for extracts from *The Natural Way to Healthful Sleep*, by Charles P. Kelly (copyright © 1961 by Charles P. Kelly); the Estate of Marie Stopes for extracts from *Sleep*, by Marie Stopes, originally published by Chatto & Windus Ltd.; *The Times*, London, for *Living with Insomnia*, by Bernard Levin, originally published in *The Times* as *Uncomfortably Awake? . . . Then I'll Begin;* Little, Brown & Co. and André Deutsch Ltd. for two poems by Ogden Nash published in *Bed Riddance* ("What, No Sheep?" copyright 1953 by Ogden Nash, "The Stilly Night" copyright © 1966 by Ogden Nash); Mrs. James Thurber and Hamish Hamilton Ltd. for extracts from "Watchers of the Night," by James Thurber, originally published in *The New Yorker* and then by Harper & Row, in *Lanterns and Lances* (copyright © 1961 by James Thurber); Mr. Roger Angell and the Viking Press for "Ainmosni," by Roger Angell, originally published in *The New Yorker*, then in *A Day in the Life of Roger Agnell* (copyright © 1970 by Roger Agnell); Mrs. Angela Mathias for the extract from *The Worst Journey in the World*, by Apsley Cherry-Garrard, published by Chatto & Windus Ltd.; Professor Ivan Morris, Walker & Co. and The Bodley Head for five puzzles from *The Pillow-Book Puzzles*, by Ivan Morris (copyright © 1969 by Ivan Morris); Mr. Edward de Bono for five puzzles originally published in the *Daily Telegraph Magazine;* and Brian W. Aldiss for "Reflections of an Ardent Insomniac," first published in *The Guardian* (copyright © Brian W. Aldiss 1972); Brandt & Brandt for "The Sleep Clinic," by Maggie Scarf (copyright © 1973 by Maggie Scarf); McGraw-Hill Book Company for an extract from *Beyond Time,* by Michel Siffre, translated by Herma Briffault (copyright © 1964 by Michel Siffre).

I am deeply grateful for the consistently cheerful help of my assistant, Anne Abel Smith.

I have reserved to the last the debt of gratitude which I owe to my wife. Being married to an insomniac often presents problems to the sleeping partner, but the insomniac spouse who talks of nothing else for a whole year and who shamelessly brings the subject up at every dinner-table conversation would strain most people's tolerance beyond bearing. I have been—and am—very lucky in my marriage.

For the idea of putting together a book on this subject, and for the title, I am indebted to my insomnia.

Contents

☆

Contents

Introduction

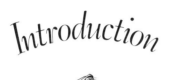

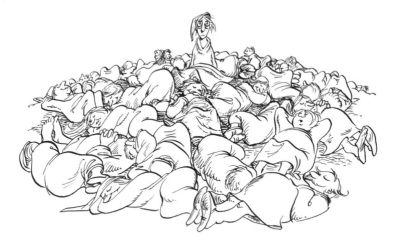

Ruminating one morning about three o'clock on the various mental exercises that I habitually employ to occupy my mind in the sleepless hours of the night, I began to wonder how other insomniacs coped with their involuntary waking states. It occurred to me how little I'd ever read on the subject. What was known about the amount of sleep the body or the mind really needs? Was there one kind of insomnia or several? Were there any cures or only palliatives? How useful—or how dangerous—were all the different kinds of drugs now on the market or available with a doctor's prescription? Or the multitude of advertised sleep-aid devices? What, indeed, was known about the nature of sleep itself, its chemistry, and that small but crucial part of sleep devoted to dreaming?

When I came to examine the literature of sleep, I realized that I had stumbled not on a pond but on an ocean of a subject. Though I had read an occasional article, I had no idea just how extensive had been the research on sleep in the last quarter of a century, and especially in the past decade. Some experts have claimed that probes into "inner space," as it is sometimes called, are likely in the end to rival in importance the spectacular successes in outer space and oceanographic research. Yet the general public knows comparatively little about the strange work of the sleep laboratories.

The assumption of this book is that fellow insomniacs will be as interested as I have been to learn more about the profound mysteries of sleep and non-sleep as well as about some of the innumerable techniques that have been devised for alleviating unwelcome wakefulness.

People who have never had a bad night's sleep in their life cannot possibly imagine the sense of martyrdom of the severe insomniac. President Truman professed not to have lost a night's sleep even in the worst crises of his Administration. In contrast, Lord Rosebery had to resign as Prime Minister of England because of his chronic insomnia. "I cannot forget 1895," he was to write eight years later. "To lie, night after night, staring wide awake, hopeless of sleep, tormented in nerves and to realise all that was going on, at which I was present, so to speak, like a disembodied spirit, to watch one's own corpse, as it were, day after day, is an experience which no sane man with a conscience would repeat."

"I feel injured by my insomnia as though I have been left out of a marvelous party everyone else enjoys and I can only watch," one insomniac correspondent wrote to me. "The desire for sleep is not unlike the desire for marriage," wrote another. "The more you want it, the less likely you are to get it." Since I started to take an interest in the subject, I have had hundreds of letters from insomniacs; this sense of envy and resentment is a characteristic reaction.

"Pity us! Oh pity us! We wakeful," wrote Rudyard Kipling. Indeed, insomniacs do lack sympathy. It's easy to see why. In the night, the long, long insomniac night, you are condemned to suffer alone; even if you have a regular bed companion, there's a limit to how much nudging and conversation making you can do to a sleeping partner who really wants to sleep. But things aren't necessarily more cheerful in the day that follows, as you drag yourself around morose and gray. If you have laryngitis (that most peaceful and congenial of ailments) or a patch over your eye or an arm in a sling, you can be sure to attract comforting responses from your neighbors and colleagues. But as an insomniac, unless you put on a histrionic pose of suffering, no one is likely to ask how you are feeling. And just try dropping into the conversation a remark like "Incidentally, I didn't sleep a wink last night" and watch the bored, heartless faces of your audience.

Some insomniacs, even when in great distress, find it very difficult to tell doctors of their sleep problems. But even when they do, they may not get much sympathy. Insomnia is one of those complaints—migraine and breast-feeding difficulties are two others—which persistently fail to get the attention they deserve from the medical profession. The trouble is that there's nothing discernibly wrong with the patient who complains he can't sleep; it's not like having boils or ulcers or a slipped disc or a straightforward case of fever which offers the doctor something palpable to treat. Moreover, insomnia isn't something simple or single: there are many different kinds. Obviously, the most familiar sort is that which stems fairly directly from a particular crisis in an individual's life: bereavement, desertion, a violent quarrel, anxiety about one's job, a car crash, exam nerves. When the cause of the stress disappears, sleep normally returns, though a severe trauma can throw a long shadow. But it is quite common for people to suffer from imaginary insomnia, having an exaggerated view of the part of the night actually spent awake, or confusing sleeping and waking because of being unable to distinguish clearly between dreams and waking thoughts. And then there is chronic or pathological insomnia, with many possible causes, sometimes buried deep in the victim's subconscious. Most doctors don't pretend to be lay analysts, and are often unable to give sufficient time to explore a patient's subconscious. Even so, it's astonishing that doctors who would insist on a careful examination before prescribing a painkiller to a patient complaining of stomach ache will nonchalantly write out a prescription for sleeping pills for the insomniac without any serious attempt at diagnosis.

Despite the explosion in sleep studies in the last twenty years, with more and more volunteers clocking in at laboratories night after night to be wired up to electroencephalograph machines, despite everything that these researches have taught us about the patterns of sleeping and dreaming, the significance of rapid eye movements, the chemistry and biology and pharmacology of sleep, the fact is that we are still not clear as to what constitutes a good night's sleep, how sleep is brought about and why it is required—and we are equally ignorant, if not more so, about the nature and incidence of insomnia. Experts of many kinds have engaged in sleep studies in recent years. The picture is one of high optimism in the late fifties and early sixties, following the discovery of rapid eye movements, and growing disappointment in recent years. As so often with scientific breakthroughs, the more optimistic claims have turned out to be unjustified, or at least premature. You could liken this research to torches dimly illuminating a vast underground cave. Thin pencils of light pierce the darkness in places, but the proportions and extent of the cavern cannot yet be fathomed.

We believe insomnia to be on the increase, but the only hard fact in a welter of speculation is that in the fifties and sixties there was an alarming increase in the consumption of sleeping pills in every advanced country of the Western world. National Health Service prescriptions for barbiturates in England and Wales doubled between 1953 and 1959; in Czechoslovakia they doubled between 1958 and 1965; in Australia they more than doubled between 1962 and 1966. American figures are even more staggering: between 1953 and 1965, the sale of drugs which soothe the nerves increased more than five times. Although barbiturates are no longer being prescribed so readily, and, in most states, are more closely regulated by law, there appears to have been little let up in the demand for sleeping pills and their like. In the United States today there are about two hundred different sedatives and tranquilizers on the market—to say nothing of the antihistamines which are marketed over the counter with "sleepy" names. We can't, of course, be sure how many pills are bought but never swallowed; a look at many people's medicine cabinets suggests that the pharmaceutical industry, like the manufacturers of mustard, make their living by what is left behind rather than what is actually consumed. Yet the statistics are certainly disturbing.

Are sleeping pills a menace? One recent U.S. report claimed that 4,000 deaths a year could be directly attributed to the abuse of nonprescription drugs, and they obviously are indirectly responsible for accidents on the roads and in industry. Many regard them as anathema, as yet another shameful crutch in an increasingly decadent society. It's also true that sleeping pills have become tainted with the evil repute of other drugs that have come into public prominence in recent years—pep pills, for example, or LSD, or, most notoriously, thalidomide. Perhaps, too, they are associated in people's minds with a host of other technological advances that now appear in a less rosy light than hitherto: chemical fertilizers, unrecyclable plastic bottles, high-rise apartments or supersonic aircraft. There are those to whom technological progress itself has become a dirty word.

Certainly the bad reputation which drugs have earned is not undeserved. The drug companies themselves have been partly responsible in their "pushing" of drugs, and doctors, too, have often been to blame for recommending pills fecklessly without knowing enough about their properties or side effects. It is only in the last ten years that people have awakened to the dangers of barbiturate addiction. Thanks to the sleep laboratories, we now know a lot about how barbiturates impair motor and psychological functions, distort the pattern of dreaming, and once having been taken regularly, provoke dire withdrawal symptoms. It is difficult to understand why it took so long for the harmful side effects of so many of these drugs to be recognized by the medical profession.

All tranquilizers and sedatives, so far discovered, disturb our regular sleep patterns, and alter the duration and intensity of our dreaming. Recently, however, a group of tranquilizers known as benzodiazepines has come to be widely used. They certainly seem a great deal safer and more effective than any comparable drugs previously available, and far better than barbiturates for treating sleep problems. It is very difficult to take an overdose of these tranquilizers, and there is not much evidence that they are addictive. Librium and Valium are the best-known brand names of the various compounds. Although usually described as tranquilizers, they could be called sedatives, too: any of the drugs in this group relax the muscles and act as a mild sedative, and are equally useful in alleviating anxiety or insomnia.

In short, not everyone who takes a sleeping pill need find it habit forming; and anti-pill crusades, like campaigns against road improvements, can go too far. We are right to be alarmed at the increase in pill taking, particularly since there are safer ways to encourage sleep, but sedatives can be immeasurably helpful in the temporary insomnia caused by a serious personal crisis. A lot of us may be walking around with crutches we don't need, but it's only a fool who refuses a crutch when he really is crippled.

At this point a reader may well ask how I came to put such a jaunty title to this book, since insomnia is obviously a serious subject which has had nothing like the medical attention it deserves. It's true that insomnia isn't much of a laughing matter (though it's inspired some of the best of Thurber and Ogden Nash); yet, having spent most of this past year reading everything I could on the subject, talking to experts, and as a result of appeals in the press and on radio, having received a huge mailbag from insomniac correspondents, I have come to the conclusion that many insomniacs worry about their complaint more than they need to and more than is good for them.

I write this, knowing perfectly well how exasperating that comment will seem to certain readers who at this moment are going through torment from their inability to sleep. It's as though (they might claim) I were to say to a man crying out for help in rough seas, "Don't worry—you're only drowning." But my remarks about exaggerated worry are not intended to apply to *all* insomniacs. A man who goes to his doctor complaining of insomnia *must* be taken seriously; insomnia is often an early warning of an impending mental breakdown, or an attempt at suicide. Doctors treat such patients lightly at their peril. Yet most insomniacs most of the time are not about to break down, and it is to this not-so-suffering majority that my remarks are chiefly addressed.

Perhaps I should put in a personal word here. When I began to take an interest in this subject, I thought of myself as a mild insomniac. I don't always get to sleep very easily, but my sleep problems usually come in the early hours of the morning: I sleep for three or four hours and then find myself uncomfortably awake for an hour or two before dropping off again until it's time to get up. I used to resent these waking hours and would toss and turn in anguish if not in anger, to the extreme boredom of my wife. It was during one of these fretful periods that I started to think how little I knew about the nature of insomnia and resolved to find out more. Almost at once I discovered two scientific facts which transformed the way in which I regarded my insomnia. The first concerned the amount of sleep the body needs: while we have been conditioned from childhood to believe that the human system requires an average of eight hours' sleep a night, the fact is that sleep needs vary *enormously* between one person and another. The second fact, equally simple, is that whatever our personal sleep requirements, they tend to diminish as we grow older—that waking more at night is a *natural* occurrence.

Like many other home truths, those two facts were blindingly obvious as soon as they had been pointed out. I then came to realize that five or six hours' sleep a night in two snatches, with an hour or two awake in between, is all that I seem to need at this stage in life to perform adequately the following day. The hangdog air that I used to assume after a series of such nights was entirely a result of my early conditioning and my ignorance of my real sleep needs.

The most important truth about the suffering of insomnia is that it is caused by worrying about lack of sleep, not lack of sleep in itself. As a result of these revelations, I now consider myself a fraudulent, or at least a former, insomniac. I still wake up for an hour or two most nights, but no longer worry as I used to. I am convinced that many other insomniacs are victims of the same self-deception and are inflating their suffering because they haven't understood or accepted that they need less sleep than they were taught to believe they needed.

In the past half-century we have shed so many taboos, social and sexual, that we are inclined to think that there are none left to bother about. But it's always easy to spot the taboos which are on their way out, and much harder to come to terms with those which still hold us in thrall. We can laugh at our mothers' hangups about feeding infants by the clock or all that agonizing over toilet training and regular bowel movements. If we are parents, we no longer worry so much about our kids finishing up what's on their plates. Yet the myth that they must be in bed by a certain hour and get a predetermined quota of sleep persists. It has conditioned my own generation, and seems likely to haunt the next as well; and it sets up tensions that can last right through one's life.

What pernicious nonsense it is! In Mediterranean countries, children play in the piazzas until far into the night, without apparent harm. Most of them will have had siestas, so their total intake of sleep is probably much the same as children elsewhere. But the important point is that the parents don't seem anxious to get them off their hands. This anxiety about our children getting their proper ration of sleep is, I suspect, something peculiar to our present society, and it is of course connected with our attitudes to children in general. Naturally there are times when a child is plainly suffering from lack of sleep and has to be pushed or coaxed off to bed because he'd never go of his own accord. But only too often when children are reluctant to be put to bed, it's because they are punishing their parents for so patently wanting them out of the way. As a parent myself, I'm uncomfortably aware how I prize that time of peace in the evening when the children are safely nested down. A child doesn't have to be particularly bright to catch on to what's happening.

Even if we're not trying to get the children off to bed in order to be unencumbered, our own conditioning inclines us to project notions about sleep requirements which may have little or nothing to do with their real sleep needs. Some children need ten hours' sleep a night, others much less. And those who are constantly being nagged to turn off the light before they are genuinely tired ("You won't be ready for school in time tomorrow morning") are obviously on their way to becoming sleep neurotics later in life.

The subject of sleep needs is surrounded by myths and shibboleths, and lacks much in the way of solid facts. On the average an adult needs about eight hours' sleep a night, but the variations are so wide that this information is of little use except in a statistical sense. There are plenty of healthy adults who, like Napoleon, manage regularly on three or four hours' sleep a night, or even less. Others, emulating Churchill, work best through much of the night, but make up for the lost hours in bed at night by catnaps during the day. Those adults who require ten or twelve hours of sleep to function at their best are no less robust than the rest of us—their recharging processes just take longer.

Even the fact that sleep needs diminish with age isn't all that clear-cut. Some elderly people sleep more, reverting to infantile patterns of sleep, with naps taken intermittently throughout the day. But the research of sleep laboratories has shown that we have fewer periods of dreaming in our later years and that we need less heavy sleep. Hence we wake more frequently in the night as we get older and are more likely to complain of insomnia.

A great many questions remain to be answered. So far, most of the sleep laboratories are used strictly for research. In the whole of the United States there are only three sleep clinics regularly treating people with sleep disorders. There are none yet in Britain. If an insomniac shows symptoms of severe mental disorder, he will probably get the treatment he needs; if not, he is likely to be offered pills or be left to his own devices.

Despite all the techniques and appliances for coping with insomnia, the secret of sleep and of unworried non-sleep would seem to depend—like pretty much everything else in life—on that Delphic prescription, "Know thyself." Although there will always be bad times in our life when our normal patterns of sleep are dislocated (and not only bad times—falling in love is just as much an enemy of sleep as passion unrequited), we are more likely to be reconciled to our nocturnal vigils if we understand what our normal sleep requirements really are.

There aren't, it seems, any definitive *cures* for insomnia, or at least no tricks or palliatives which can be guaranteed to work for all insomniacs all the time. But I have begun to wonder whether some of the so-called victims aren't (to use Louis Auchincloss' memorable phrase) injustice collectors—people secretly or subconsciously enjoying their suffering. In my own nocturnal waking, for example, I'm aware that a particular problem may be responsible for keeping me awake—worrying about work, for instance, or mentally drafting yet another rude letter to our builder. By an effort of will I could disperse this unproductive traffic and perform some exercise of relaxation; I could, but I don't care to. Like relief for so many other psychosomatic disorders, the solution for insomnia—if we really want it—usually lies in ourselves. If my title has an inner meaning, it is in the nature of a gentle put-down. The full title, including the suppressed afterthought, would read: *Insomniacs of the world, goodnight. You have nothing to lose but your plaints.*

I have included in this book some bedtime reading for the insomniac who has tried and given up on the known recipes for sleep and is still wide awake. Different people want different kinds of nighttime sustenance—in reading as much as in food or drink or sex. Some like to be soothed, others entertained, and others again to have their minds stretched but in directions remote from their habitual cares.

Even if you're not reading, staying awake need not be a tribulation. I don't want to sound like Norman Vincent Peale, but sleeplessness can be used positively as well as reacted to negatively. People often talk about "sleeping on a problem," but not sleeping may be even better: dilemmas which seem insuperable during the tension of the day often resolve themselves when the body is at rest and there's no distracting din from the outside world. Here is how one correspondent put the case for wakefulness:

When the occasional night of insomnia turned into regular routine, I stopped cursing the darkness. As one of the night people, I realized I was among the select. The days are crowded with the millions competing with each other for quiet areas of existence. We, however, have the world to ourselves. There's a feeling of one-upmanship about being awake when almost everyone is asleep. There's a consciousness about being alive, smelling the night air, listening to the house respond to wind and rain—that can't really be done in the daytime when the routine of existence obtrudes. Whatever your life's problems are, they cease for a time, for the solution that requires the involvement of a second person must be delayed.

Night-time is perhaps the only time when you really face yourself and find out what you are and why. If you cannot be good company for yourself, how then do others look on you? For, as Aiken says, "Separate we come, Separate go. And this be it known is all that we know."

Some people obviously find facing themselves the worst of all possible ordeals; they'll grab at anything—drugs or the telephone, all-night radio or an unputdownable thriller—to avoid the confrontation. The same people may also, without realizing it, be funking sleep for fear of troubled dreams. But if we want to know ourselves, there's no better time to practice that most difficult task than in the silent hours of the night.

I draw attention to the inadequately recognized benefits of wakefulness, but would not deny that sleep, if you can get it, is preferable, and that some regular amount of sleep is essential for mental and physical health. If this book assists readers to enjoy better sleep, it will have fulfilled its purpose. But even if none of the recommended remedies or treatments help, I still feel it possible to praise insomnia rather than curse it. Blessed are the owls, for they shall inhabit the mystery and magic of the night. Blessed are the larks, for they shall inherit the dawn.

H.R.

Part One: Exploring Sleep

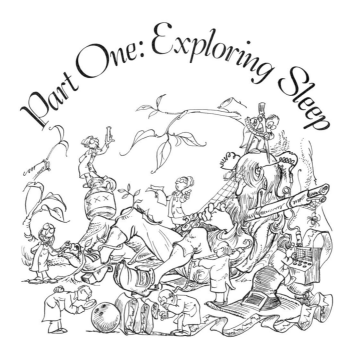

Anecdotes and Aphorisms

Insomnia never kills a man until he kills himself.

—Axel Munthe

*   *   *

So convincing were these dreams of lying awake that he awoke from them each morning in complete exhaustion and fell right back to sleep.

—Joseph Heller

*   *   *

Mulla Nasrudin was walking through the streets at midnight. The Watchman asked: "What are you doing out so late, Mulla?" "My sleep has disappeared and I am looking for it."

—Idries Shah

*   *   *

Sleep is the most moronic fraternity in the world, with the heaviest dues and crudest rituals.

—Vladimir Nabokov

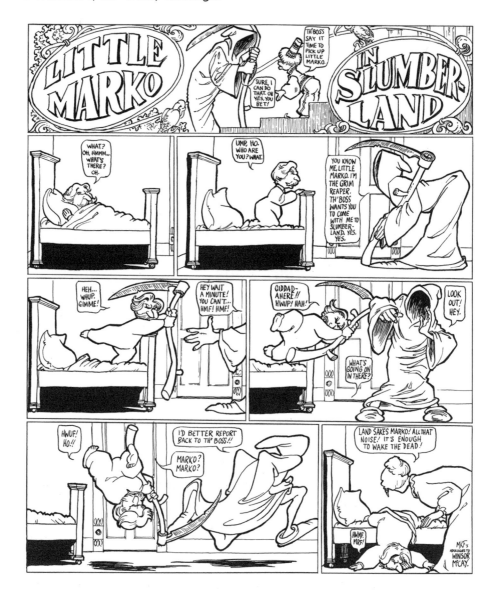

"No wonder you've got insomnia. All you ever do is sleep."
—Peter de Vries

*   *   *

When I came to be called up for my army medical, I told the examining medical officer that I suffered from insomnia. He was delighted. "You'll find insomnia very useful in the army," he said. He was quite right. I did.
—An anonymous correspondent

*   *   *

No small art is it to sleep: it is necessary to keep awake all day for that purpose.
—Nietzsche

*   *   *

He's such a terrible insomniac: he even dreams he's awake.
—Jewish joke

*   *   *

Mark Twain warned his friends against going to bed—"so many people die there."

*   *   *

I am always curious about how people fall asleep. I recently asked Sam Goldwyn, who is in his eighties, what he did about sleep.

He replied, "I take a dull book to bed."

I said to my friend S. N. Behrman, "If we knew the name of that dull book, we could clean up."
—Oscar Levant

How We Sleep and Why We Sleep

It is a commonplace if engrossing thought that nine tenths of all scientists who have ever lived are alive at the present time. But if we were discussing the study of sleep, the ratio would be even more staggering: hardly any sleep research had been done before the beginning of the present century and virtually all our present knowledge about the physiology and chemistry of sleep derives from work done in the last forty years, mostly in the past two decades. Considering how large a part of human and animal existence is spent in the profound darkness of the unconscious, it is extraordinarily difficult to understand why this rich seam of a subject has taken so long to be explored and developed.

As Archimedes, according to legend, founded the science of hydrostatics by observing the displacement of water when he stepped into his bath, and Newton formulated the laws of gravitation after watching the fall of an apple, so the key observation in the science of sleep also came about in a serendipitous fashion. One day in April 1952, at the University of Chicago, a young physiology graduate named Eugene Aserinsky noticed that people asleep had periods during the night when, for several minutes at a time, their eyes were in rapid motion. Over the centuries, a multitude of insomniacs, enviously watching the slumber of their spouses, may have noticed the same phenomenon and not given it a second thought. Aserinsky, however, did not make his discovery by direct observation: he was using an electroencephalograph (or EEG for short) —a machine which picks up, amplifies and records on graph paper tiny alterations in voltage from different parts of the body. At first he refused to believe the graph, preferring to think that the machine had broken. It was only when he himself looked at the sleeper and found that he could actually see the eyeballs in motion beneath the lids that he became convinced of the genuineness of the evidence.

The discovery of these rapid eye movements (or REMs, as they are now usually called) became doubly significant when it was found that sleepers disturbed during a REM period almost invariably reported dreams. The following year Aserinsky, together with a colleague in his Chicago laboratories, Nathaniel Kleitman,* reported their findings in *Science* under the forbidding title "Regularly Occurring Periods of Eye Motility and Concomitant Phenomena During Sleep." A significant passage ran:

> Of twenty-seven interrogations during ocular motility, twenty revealed detailed dreams. Of twenty-three interrogations during ocular inactivity, nineteen disclosed complete failure of recall.

For practical purposes, sleep studies may be said to have started with the publication of this article in 1953, and since then they have burgeoned all over the world. It is one of the relatively few cases on record of a scientific breakthrough opening up an entirely new field of research. Here is how Frederick

---

*Kleitman, if anyone, deserves the title of founding father of sleep research. His major work, *Sleep and Wakefulness* (revised edition, 1963), is by far the most comprehensive book in the field, though I agree with the sleep scientist who described it to me as "the most somnifacient book ever: will cure any insomniac."

Snyder, research psychiatrist at the National Institute of Mental Health, described its significance:

> In the Upanishads of ancient India it is written that existence takes three forms, the one here in this world, another in the other world, and a third in the world of dreaming. By the second half of the 20th century scientific views of nature had nothing to say of the other world, and, with the singular and therefore highly suspect exception of psychiatry, they were equally silent about the realm of dreaming. If our era will be remembered for first exploring the other world of outer space, it may be just as important that it produced the first concerted assault upon the secret workings of the brain whence comes our inner world of nightly visions . . . It is now apparent that human dreaming is the subjective aspect of an extremely substantial, predictable, universal and basic biological function. The physiological characteristics of this phenomenon prove so distinctive that I consider it a third state of earthly existence, the rapid eye movement or REM state, which is at least as different from sleeping and waking as each is from the other.*

The excitement was understandable, even if, with hindsight, somewhat premature. We now know a good deal about the mechanics of sleep and dreaming and the daily rhythms of the body, but why we sleep, why we dream—these are still crucial questions that lack confident answers. "It is seldom in the history of physiology," wrote the distinguished French sleep scientist Michel Jouvet in 1967, "that a phenomenon has been analyzed with such accuracy, without this analysis revealing its possible functions." Seven years later, its functions are still not apparent. Like the black holes in space, which so intrigue and baffle astronomers, sleep cannot be probed directly, though most of us acknowledge almost every night of our lives the astounding strength of its gravitational pull.

What are these two different kinds of sleep—orthodox and REM? One sort of answer can be given with great precision, thanks to the electroencephalo-

*From "Towards an Evolutionary Theory of Dreaming," in the *American Journal of Psychiatry* (August 1966).

The Stages of a Normal Sleep Cycle

STAGE	BRAIN WAVES	BEHAVIOR AND SENSATIONS	DEPTH OF SLEEP	PHYSIOLOGICAL CHANGES	DREAMS
The threshold of sleep (alpha) and relaxed wakefulness	An even rhythm (the alpha rhythm), 9–12 cycles per second	Serene relaxation, no concentrated thought	Perceptions slowing down		Fragments of thought
. . .the myoclonic jerk	. . .tiny bursts of electrical activity in the brain	. . .a sudden spasm, causing the body to jerk	Momentary arousal		
I	Small and pinched, irregular and rapidly changing	Sometimes a floating sensation, drifting with idle thoughts and dreams	Can still be awakened easily, and will insist has not been asleep	Muscles relaxing, pulse growing even, breathing becoming regular, temperature falling	Images and thoughtlike fragments
II	Growing larger, quick bursts, resembling wire spindle	If eyes are open, will not see	May be awakened with a modest sound	Eyes roll slowly from side to side	Some thoughtlike fragments and low-intensity dreams

STAGE	BRAIN WAVES	BEHAVIOR AND SENSATIONS	DEPTH OF SLEEP	PHYSIOLOGICAL CHANGES	DREAMS
III	Large, slow waves —one per second	Removed from the waking world	Takes louder noise to awaken	Muscles relaxed, breathing even; heart rate slowed, temperature declining, muscles relaxed, blood pressure dropping	Rarely recalled
IV (delta)	Very large, slow waves (delta waves) that trace a jagged pattern	Period of beginning sleepwalking, or bed wetting	The deepest sleep, most difficult to awaken	Even breathing, heart rate, blood pressure; body temperature slowly falling	Poor recall makes this seem like a dreamless oblivion most of the time; rare nightmares
REM	Irregular and small —resembles those of waking	Rapid eye movements (REMs) as if watching	Hard to bring to the surface and reality	Lies limp, chin muscles slack; penile erections; increased gastric secretions in ulcer patients; fluctuating blood pressure; irregular pulse, respiration; twitching of fingers and toes	Very vivid dreams 85 percent of the time

The entire cycle is repeated roughly every 90 minutes, or about four or five times in a normal night.
Stage IV is most protracted in early part of the night. REM dreams grow more vivid as the night progresses.

graph. Researchers have employed the EEG to chart all kinds of physiological changes that take place during sleep: the frequency and amplitude of the rhythms of the brain, blood pressure, pulse, respiration, body temperature and muscle tone. A wide cross section of humanity—male and female, day-old infants and octogenarians, sound sleepers and insomniacs, athletes and jet pilots, drug addicts, schizoids and manic-depressives—have been wired up to EEG machines, sometimes for many nights at a stretch, and the results analyzed in minutest detail. The EEG has also been used extensively to record the sleep of animals—birds, reptiles and mammals. Since one volunteer in a single night produces some 700 yards of record, the total consumption of paper in all this research must run into many thousands of miles. But we now know a massive amount about the "how" of sleep.

Sleep scientists have somewhat arbitrarily divided the course of orthodox sleep into four successive stages (see table). Before the onset of sleep, you will notice that there is a threshold period as we lie relaxed, with our eyes normally closed, waiting for sleep to overtake us. It is during this phase that our brain waves will be registering a frequency of about 9–12 cycles a second, showing on the EEG a distinctive formation known as the alpha rhythm. The alpha waves have acquired importance recently because of their use in biofeedback therapy (see pp. 59 ff.). Sometimes, very shortly before we finally fall asleep, we may be momentarily startled by a phenomenon known as the myoclonic jerk, a sudden spasm which feels as though our heart has missed a beat. Then sleep takes over.

Every sleeping night of our lives, we repeat the same pattern of descent through these four stages—our muscles slowly becoming more relaxed, our pulse and breathing more even and our temperature falling. The EEG waves will change, becoming gradually larger and slower until they reach Stage IV, often called the delta stage, at 1–3 cycles a second, at which point our sleep is at its most profound. Then, quite suddenly and dramatically, after about ninety minutes, we enter our REM period. At once our EEG pattern becomes irregular and fast, resembling a waking state, and our eyes move rapidly; a man's penis may become erect. Almost certainly, if we were now to be awakened (though it is as hard to wake a sleeper in REM as it is in Stage IV), we would report a dream. The REM state will continue for about ten or fifteen minutes. Then once more we make our gradual descent through the four stages. The same cycle is likely to be repeated at similar intervals four or five times during the night, though we spend less time later in the night in stages III and IV, and our REM periods will probably last somewhat longer.

One remarkable feature of this nightly journey up and down the staircase of consciousness is its constancy. Unless our sleep processes are interfered with —as may happen if we take certain drugs or after heavy drinking—we always experience these two states of sleep, orthodox and REM.* In healthy adults, orthodox sleep usually occupies about three quarters of the total sleep period, and REM the remaining quarter. Orthodox invariably precedes REM. We always enjoy more deep (stages III and IV) sleep in the early part of the sleep period. The length of the complete cycle hardly varies between 90 and 110 minutes. And the same constant features are found among almost all verte-brates—reptiles, birds and mammals—although the length of the sleep cycle varies according to the size of the species. Even the primitive opossum shows distinctive orthodox and REM periods. Only in one very primitive mammal, the spiny anteater, has the REM state not been found; it would seem that the two states of sleep must have been laid down very early in the evolutionary process.

Here are a few more significant facts about our sleep habits. Adults, as we

~~~~~~

*Perhaps at this point I should warn the reader that if he pursues sleep studies, he will come across a number of different terms for the same phenomena. Orthodox sleep is often known as NREM or non-REM or non-rapid-eye-movement sleep or S (for synchronized EEG) sleep. REM is also known as D (for desynchro-nized EEG or dreaming) sleep or as paradoxical sleep (PS). The paradox is that by the EEG criteria, sleep appears to be light during REM, though the muscles are at their most relaxed, and as we have seen, it is as hard to arouse a sleeper in REM as it is in Stage IV.

know, normally sleep seven or eight hours a night (slightly less as they grow older), and newborn infants between sixteen and eighteen hours. But while young adults spend only a quarter of their sleep in dream periods and their REM periods diminish with age, infants spend at least *half* their sleep time in REM, and preliminary studies in animals suggest that the uterine fetus may have an even higher REM percentage. Whatever function or functions sleep serves, it is clearly more required in the very young—and the REM sleep in this phase has an even greater importance than orthodox sleep.

By far the most popular kind of sleep experiment (though "popular" may not be the happiest term in this context) has been in sleep deprivation. In order to discover the function of an organ, it is a traditional routine in medical science to remove it from a laboratory animal and see what happens. Sleep-deprivation experiments have been carried out with many kinds of animals, and one fact is clear: if they are deprived of sleep long enough, they die. Young dogs, for instance, die in less than a week, and adult dogs in about a fortnight.

But there have also been innumerable sleep-deprivation experiments with humans. Of course we all know in crude terms what happens when we deprive someone of sleep; it is one of the commonest tortures in psychological warfare, though the practice predates modern psychology. No doubt man dies too if the torture is maintained for a sufficient period. No statistics, one is happy to say, are available from the sleep laboratories on this point, but there is a great deal of evidence about the changes in behavior that follow a prolonged sleep loss. Insomniacs will not need to be told that the general effect of loss of sleep is to make the subject more angry or irritable than he would be otherwise, with a greater difficulty in focusing his attention. In extreme cases—after four or more days of total deprivation—there is likely to be a tendency toward a general personality collapse, with visual and auditory hallucinations. But few insomniacs are likely to reach this stage. Bad sleepers are much given to self-deception; they may claim that they never slept a wink, but this is almost never the case. Moreover, the time it takes to recover from sleep loss is comparatively short—comparative, that is, to the loss. A person may suffer several nights of sleep loss in a row, but one good night's sleep, perhaps an hour or two longer than usual, will see him fully recovered.

One of the more interesting kinds of sleep-deprivation experiments are those concerned with subsequent performance. There are many variations of such experiments, but the basic pattern is for groups of volunteers to be deprived in turn of differing amounts of sleep, and the effects tested the following day by a series of rigorous tasks. You might think that loss of sleep would be reflected in any work undertaken the next day, but Dr. R. T. Wilkinson, of the Medical Research Council's Applied Psychology Unit in Cambridge, England, one of the leading experts in this field, has shown that it is in fact only the long, boring, repetitive task—endless counting of simple sums, for instance—which will show up the difference between an 8-hour and a 4-hour sleeper, and that as soon as the subject's interest is aroused, sleep loss tends to make relatively little difference. Of course the subject's motivation can affect these results. "Different people," says Wilkinson, "have a different tolerance for sleep deprivation, and react to it emotionally in varying ways. Some will be challenged by stress and will achieve normal performances, not necessarily because they are unaffected by sleep deprivation, but because they can compensate by extra effort, though what the long-term physiological cost of this is we do not know. One thing we have learned is that if people want to maintain normal performances, it's surprising how well they can." In Wilkinson's most recent experiments, performance is seen to be only significantly impaired when a volunteer suffers two successive nights of five hours' sleep or less, or a single night with less than two hours' sleep.

There is an obvious moral here for the insomniac. Students faced with an important exam frequently sleep badly the night before, and worry that it will affect their results. Wilkinson's findings show that such anxieties are often unnecessary, that only repeated and exceptionally disturbed nights will damage the student's chances; a bank clerk, whose work is largely routine, is more likely to lose his job because of sleeplessness than the student to fail his exams.

We could take the moral further and ask how often, in the torment of a bad night, we have declared that we would be good for nothing the next day, and then surprised ourselves by discovering that, though a bit groggy, we were in fact able to perform in a perfectly adequate way? In other words, how much of our insomnia—our *worry* about not getting enough sleep—is really necessary? If we are still able to perform effectively despite difficulties in getting to sleep, broken nights or early awakenings, our neuroses about getting sufficient sleep should be greatly eased. Moreover, if we accept Wilkinson's criterion of a good night's sleep as that which enables us to perform effectively the following day, may we not have a new and valuable test of the efficacy or otherwise of a sleeping pill? Many of us have found that we were far more confused the day after taking a pill than we ever were after a night of tossing and turning without benefit of sedation. Could it be that the cure is sometimes worse than the ailment?

Before we leave the subject of sleep deprivation, I should say something about the experiments designed to deprive an individual of one state of sleep while leaving him in full enjoyment of the other. These experiments are important because they throw light on the respective functions of the two kinds of sleep, but they are fraught with practical problems; in particular, it has proved very difficult to deprive a man of his orthodox sleep while leaving him in possession of his dream state.* However, a recent technique has succeeded in depriving subjects of their Stage IV, their deep slow-wave sleep, without too many awakenings or too great a reduction in their total sleep time. The results of various experiments, though not conclusive, may be summarized as follows: if we lose our Stage IV sleep, we tend to suffer nothing more than a general lethargy the following day, but if we have our dream periods interfered with, we are more likely to find that our capacity to focus attention on a given task

***

*Indeed, the whole business of sleep deprivation is fraught with difficulties, largely because subjects can so easily take a micro-nap without the investigator being able to catch them at it. One well-known sleep researcher, W. L. Webb, surveying the field, was forced ruefully to conclude: "The effect of sleep deprivation is to make the subject fall asleep."

will be diminished, and in general that our mechanisms of learning and memory will be impaired.

Another kind of sleep research is concerned with investigating the differences between those who habitually need a lot of sleep and those who regularly get by on much less. Among many experiments with long and short sleepers, one of the most interesting was that carried out by Ernest L. Hartmann of the Sleep and Dream Laboratory at Boston State Hospital. Hartmann chose two groups of people who represented extremes of sleep duration—the long sleepers averaging 8 1/2 hours a night and the short ones about 5 1/2 hours. In other respects both groups, so far as questionnaires and selection interviews could show, were normal enough—none of his volunteers were taking drugs and none had any particular complaint about his sleep habits.

When these two groups were given EEG tests, a startling fact emerged. Despite the great difference in total sleep time between the long and the short sleepers, they all spent almost exactly the same amount of time in slow-wave (stages III and IV) sleep. The difference was largely made up in REM time —an average of 121 minutes in the long sleepers, compared with 65 in the short, and the long sleepers also spent more time in Stage II. Interestingly, the long sleepers spent more time awake during the night, and felt less refreshed in the morning.

On the evidence of this experiment, it appears that there is a fairly constant human need for a given amount of slow-wave sleep, but a greatly varying need for REM.

But Hartmann did not leave his experiment there; he went on to subject his volunteers to a series of psychological tests. This is how he describes the difference he found between the short and the long sleepers:*

～～～～～～～～～～～～～～～～～～～～～～～～～～～～～～～

*From *The Functions of Sleep* (Yale University Press, 1973). I am greatly indebted to Hartmann for much in the present chapter, and I recommend his book warmly to anyone interested in learning more about sleep studies. It is the only book available which collates, connects and interprets the latest findings over the whole field of sleep research.

The short sleepers as a group were efficient, energetic, ambitious persons who tended to work hard and to keep busy. They were relatively sure of themselves, socially adept, decisive and were satisfied with themselves and their lives. They had few complaints about their life situations, or about politics and the state of the world. Their social and political views were somewhat conformist, and they wished to appear very normal and "all-American." They were extroverted and definitely not "worriers"; they seldom left themselves time to sit down and think about problems—in fact, several of them, on being asked what they did in times of stress or worry, made statements such as "I never let my worries go to my head." They seemed relatively free from psychopathology; but insofar as there was pathology, it consisted of a tendency to avoid problems by keeping busy and by denial, which in some cases approached hypomania.

The long sleepers were a less easily definable group than the short sleepers. They worked at a large range of employments; several of them were "eternal students"; and they tended to be nonconformist and critical in their social and political views. The long sleepers were more uncomfortable in many ways than the short sleepers; they complained of a variety of minor aches and pains and also complained about the laboratory. Although none of them were seriously ill psychiatrically, most had mild or moderate neurotic problems. Some were overtly anxious, some showed considerable inhibition in aggressive and sexual functioning, and some were mildly depressed. They appeared, in general, not very sure of themselves, their career choices or their life styles; however, several appeared to be artistic and creative persons. A few were aware that they sometimes used sleep as an escape when reality was unpleasant. Most of them valued sleep highly and felt it important to obtain the proper amount of sleep every night. Overall they were definitely "worriers" who did let their problems "go to their heads." The long sleepers could be seen as constantly "reprogramming" themselves as opposed to the relatively "preprogrammed" short sleepers. Thus definite differences were found between the two groups; in a few words, the short sleepers tended to be "non-worriers" or "preprogrammed," while the long sleepers were "worriers" or "reprogrammers."

What conclusions can be drawn from these two profiles? Hartmann suggests that certain life styles or certain personalities require more sleep than others, and particularly more REM sleep, and he finds confirmation of this view in considering some of the great men in history who are known to have been either very long or very short sleepers. Napoleon and Edison belong to the latter group, having regularly got by with between four and six hours' sleep a night. (Short sleepers are fond of quoting Edison's dogmatic, and utterly unscientific, assertion: "Most people overeat 100% and oversleep 100% . . . That extra 100% makes them unhealthy and inefficient. The person who sleeps eight or ten hours a night is never fully asleep and never fully awake . . .") Einstein, on the other hand, was a long sleeper, as have been many other creative geniuses in science and the arts. Possibly short sleepers are men of strong will power who have trained themselves to survive on less sleep—a point of view much favored by short sleepers—but the evidence that people can deliberately cut down on their sleep needs in any significant way is thin. It seems more likely that there are these two different types with markedly different sleep requirements: effective, practical persons (top business executives, applied scientists, political leaders) in the short-sleep category, and more worried but also more creative and less conventional people in the long-sleep camp.

Further confirmation of the view that sleep needs vary according to personality and life style comes from another Hartmann experiment, this time with variable sleepers—people who have a generally stable sleep pattern, but who at times notice that their sleep requirements have altered. It was found that people needed more sleep at times of stress, depression or a change in occupation or when there was a need for increased mental effort. Some women needed more sleep in premenstrual periods. People with periodic weight problems needed more sleep when they were trying to lose weight, as did those suffering bereavement or the breakup of an important emotional relationship.

Decreased sleep needs, on the other hand, were associated with times when things were going particularly well for a person. While undergoing independent psychoanalysis, five doctors were surprised to find that they needed less sleep, presumably because analysis was relieving them of anxieties and internal conflicts. Some people who engaged in transcendental meditation also noticed that they needed an hour or two less sleep at night when they started meditating regularly. Another group reporting less need for sleep comprised a number of professional men who were retired. Their workload had previously been demanding, and they had all expected, wrongly as it turned out, that they would be sleeping longer when the strain lifted.

Many insomniacs, reading the portrait of a characteristic long sleeper or reflecting on the circumstances which increase the sleep needs of a variable sleeper, will feel that their own personal life style or personality was being described. Hartmann had in fact taken some pains to exclude insomniacs from his experiments: the long sleepers in the first experiment were all stable long sleepers, and the variable sleepers in the second experiment were only those who felt that their sleep *requirement* was increased or decreased—not those who slept less because they couldn't get the sleep they wanted. So it would be wrong to equate long sleepers with poor sleepers. Yet there clearly is a connection, emphasized by the fact that long sleepers in the first experiment woke more frequently in the night and claimed to feel less refreshed the following morning. Long sleepers could be well-compensated insomniacs—people who tend to sleep poorly but make up for it by spending longer over their sleep— but there is no evidence that long sleepers as such are in any way poor or inefficient sleepers. They take the same amount of stages III and IV sleep as the short sleeper, and simply seem to require more time in REM. It would appear more likely, therefore, that insomniacs are inefficient long sleepers or long sleepers *manqués*. Chronic insomniacs belong by temperament to those who regularly need above-average REM sleep, and temporary or periodic insomniacs are those who require more REM sleep from time to time—because of stress or bereavement or similar circumstances—yet find it difficult to take that extra REM sleep when they need it.

To discover a possible explanation for the insomniac's inefficient sleep, we need to look at another kind of experiment, one comparing groups of good and poor sleepers. In 1963, at the Sleep Laboratory of the University of Chicago, Lawrence J. Monroe selected thirty-two mild but healthy insomniacs and matched them by age, education, physique and profession with a second group of so-called good sleepers. Both groups filled out a questionnaire before being given the routine EEG treatment in the sleep laboratory. The good sleepers claimed to fall asleep on an average within seven minutes of turning off the light, the poor sleepers figured it took them an hour. The good sleepers believed that they hardly ever woke in the night—perhaps once in two weeks; the poor sleepers recalled nighttime wakings at least three times a week.

The results were revealing in a number of ways. For a start, while the good sleepers were absolutely correct about the time it took them to drop off, the poor sleepers were way off the mark—on an average it took them only about fifteen minutes to drop off instead of the alleged hour, and that despite the strangeness of the laboratory bedroom, the electrodes attached to their scalp, face and feet, not to mention a tiny thermometer in their rectum. On the other hand, the poor sleepers *under*estimated the number of times they woke during the night. Insomniacs are not consistent in their hypochrondria!

The EEG records were particularly significant. The good sleepers spent 24 percent of their time in REM, the poor sleepers only 15 percent—repeatedly waking up just at the beginning of a REM period as though wanting to deprive themselves of dreams. The good sleepers followed a regular 90–100 minute cycle in their orthodox and REM phases, but the poor sleepers took most of their delta sleep in the early part of the night and spent the second half of the night in irregular sleep cycles, with longer periods in stages I and II, much closer therefore to the threshold of arousal.

The body-temperature curves, taken from the rectal thermometer, were perhaps the most interesting of all the EEG results. The body temperature is one of the most reliable indicators of our internal clock—the circadian (or 24-hour) rhythm of sleeping and waking. The body temperature normally falls by one or two degrees at night and rises again in the morning to a plateau on which it stays until the evening. The low-temperature point at night is sometimes called the dead spot: it is usually the time when sick people die and when those who have to work through the night perform at their most inefficient. In Monroe's experiment, the temperature of the good sleepers followed the usual rhythm: it showed a marked decline at bedtime and fell to its nadir in the early hours of the morning; it began to rise an hour or two before the good sleepers awoke, and was normal by the time they got up. The temperature of the poor sleepers, in contrast, declined less, continued to fall throughout the night, and was still falling when it was time to get up.

We still know very little about our circadian rhythms, or body time, as it is sometimes called. It is one of the fields of study from which much is expected in the next decade. But it is reasonable to think, on the evidence provided by Monroe's experiment, that in its mystery lies some kind of answer to the insomniac's distress—that the insomniac, in some way we do not yet understand, is not properly synchronized with life, and that the irregularities of his sleep cycle are a reflection of some fault in the mechanism of his internal clock. Body-time theories also help to explain the phenomena of "larks" and "owls." Many poor sleepers wish that they could go to bed later and rise later (or the other way around) than is socially or occupationally acceptable; it may well be that their body time is lagging behind or is in advance of clock time. Body time may also explain the strange success of the controversial therapy known as electrosleep (see Chapter 5): it could be that electric stimulation of the brain acts as a resynchronizer of the internal rhythms which are out of kilter, that it serves to realign a person with his environment.

Is it fair to attribute to insomniacs some fault in their constitutional make-up? The word "fault" is a loaded one. It is only recently that we have learned not to attribute to women or to homosexuals an inferior or defective status, and it may be that we should watch our language in the context of sleep patterns, too. I was put in mind of this by reading a well-known passage by Churchill about his sleeping habits:

I have had recourse to a method of life which greatly extended my daily capacity for work. I always went to bed for at least one hour as early as possible in the afternoon and exploited to the full my happy gift of falling almost immediately into deep sleep. By this means I was able to press a day and a half's work into one. Nature had not intended mankind to work from eight in the morning to midnight without the refreshment of blessed oblivion which, even if it lasts only twenty minutes, is sufficient to renew all the vital forces. I regretted having to send myself to bed like a child every afternoon, but I was rewarded by being able to work through the night until two or even later—sometimes much later—in the morning, and begin the new day between eight and nine o'clock. This routine I observed throughout the war, and I commend it to others if and when they find it necessary for a long spell to get the last scrap out of the human structure.

When we know a little more about sleep than we do at present, we may well discover that there are optimal hours for certain kinds of mental or physical activity other than those which our present social setup allocates to such tasks, or that, as with Churchill, certain constitutions demand a different circadian rhythm from the norm. Some variable sleepers can work through several nights at a stretch, and then rest and recover for forty-eight hours. To say that these people have a faulty mechanism is to beg a whole lot of difficult questions.

Theories about body rhythms may tell us, admittedly in a rather cloudy way, how insomniacs come to be out of step with their more fortunate neighbors, but we still need to explain, if we can, exactly what it is that insomniacs are missing out on. If we are right in calling insomniacs inefficient long sleepers, it would seem likely that they are losing out on REM. But we still need to grapple with the central questions: Exactly what function does REM sleep serve, and is it different in kind from the function of orthodox sleep?

To help us in this inquiry, we now need to turn to yet another field of sleep research—that part devoted to studying the changes in sleep patterns with age. As we know, the newborn child needs a great deal of sleep—about eighteen hours a day—with half of that spent in REM. The total amount of sleep and the proportion spent in REM fall during the first ten to twenty years, and then level out to a plateau, falling again in the latter years of a person's life. In considering the effect of depriving people of REM, we noticed that it seemed particularly to affect the mechanisms of learning and memory. It seems reasonable to suppose, therefore, that there is a direct connection between the need for a great deal of REM in the early years and the process of acquiring and absorbing new knowledge and experiences (with all its attendant psychic stress) which are at their zenith during that period. As we advance into old age, we need to acquire less knowledge and are likely to be leading less stressful lives —hence the fall in REM in later years.

I owe to Hartmann a further insight into the possible function of sleep— and also, I believe, an insight into the nature of insomnia—from pioneer work he has done on the psychology of tiredness. Hartmann has identified two distinct patterns of tiredness: one following a day of purely physical activity, and the other an exhausting day of intellectual and/or emotional effort. The table on the next page, using the language of psychoanalysis, gives the significant features of what Hartmann calls Tiredness 1 and Tiredness 2.

Hartmann is careful to use the word "hypothesize" in his all-important bottom line. We are indeed here in the area of speculation, and touching, moreover, on one of the most controversial issues in present-day sleep studies: whether orthodox, or at least slow-wave orthodox, sleep has a more important recuperative function than REM. If Hartmann is right, sleep has an essential restorative function—as common sense has always told us it must have—but there are separable requirements for the two states of sleep. Slow-wave sleep, the deeper and probably most intensive part of our orthodox sleep, has a physically restorative function; we need more of it after active exercise, after pain or after physical injury. The restorative function of REM, on the other hand, is more connected with the ability to focus attention, especially the ability to focus attention on one item while ignoring others; with maintaining a mood of optimism and self-confidence; and with successful emotional adapta-

	TIREDNESS 1	TIREDNESS 2
ROUGH DESIGNATION	"PHYSICAL"	"MENTAL"
Typically follows	a day of physical activity, sport, or mixed physical-intellectual activity without worry or anxiety	a day of emotional stress or a day of hard, not entirely pleasant, intellectual work or intellectual plus emotional work
Muscles	Usually relaxed	Often tense
Physical symptoms	None	Sometimes headache, eye strain, or cramped or tense feelings in various muscles
Affective tone	Neutral or pleasant	Neutral or often unpleasant
Sleep onset	Rapid, easy	Sometimes slow, difficult
Mental changes (adult)	No definite changes	Discomfort, irritability, anger, lack of energy, inability to concentrate, loss of social adaptiveness, loss of ability for careful patterning or long-term planning
Mental changes (children)	No definite changes	Regression, loss of superego, emergence of naked anger or hostility, temper tantrums, "too tired to get to sleep"
Metapsychological formulation	No change	Wearing out of the most recently developed or most subtle ego mechanisms; wearing out of secondary process; emergence of drive and impulses, especially anger
Hypothesized relationship to sleep	Represents a "need" for orthodox sleep	Represents a "need" for REM sleep

tion to our environment. We need more REM sleep after days of stress or intense new learning, especially if that new learning is in itself stressful.

I offer Dr. Hartmann's conclusion, which I find intrinsically plausible, aware that I have done some severe injustice to his case through compression and omission. In particular, I have left out one of the main pillars on which he rests his arguments: the evidence from the study of the chemistry of sleep (which is unfortunately too technical to discuss here).

I am also aware that I have said nothing about the chief alternative theories as to the function of sleep, particularly the evolutionary ones, which look more closely than Hartmann does at sleep phenomena in animals. Frederick Snyder, for instance, asks how the purposes of survival can be served by the intervals of nervous excitation (REM) which punctuate the sleep of all mammals. Snyder suggests that REM serves a "sentinel" function, achieving brief but periodic awakenings and preparing the organism for immediate fight or flight; it provides maximum security from external danger compatible with minimum disturbance to the continuity of sleep. In a variant of this theory Ray Meddis, of Bedford College, London, suggests that sleep is characterized by the principle of immobility—that its chief function is the conservation of energy. Only a small part of the twenty-four hours need be spent in food gathering or other activities essential for the survival of the species; sleep is a biologically reasonable occupation for the remaining hours. In effect, sleep takes over when we have nothing better to do. It exists solely to provide the evolutionary advantages of immobility; it may serve purposes of detoxicification and rest in humans as well, but these are secondary functions. "There is no evidence that these needs would not be satisfied merely by rest, without recourse to the massive and complex alterations required by sleep . . . It is an inescapable consequence of the evolutionary approach that sleep is no longer necessary in civilised man."

I agree that Hartmann is on weak ground when his theories are applied to mammals other than man. The gorilla, for instance, does not need to engage in any great physical exertion to gather his food, since it is scattered liberally over the floor of the equatorial forests; yet the gorilla sleeps for fourteen hours a night and takes a three-hour siesta in the afternoon as well. And what function does REM serve with a gorilla? All mammals have their REM periods, mice as well as men; the more complex and flexible species have no more REM than the rest. Hartmann suggests, not very confidently, that the higher, more developed species may require more of the restoration provided by sleep, but can also obtain it more efficiently per minute of time.

Hartmann's theory may not be watertight, but it seems to me a great deal closer to the truth than any other theories at present available. I cannot be convinced by the argument that claims it would not matter if man used no sleep at all. The evidence from the sleep deprivation experiments seems to me quite irrefutable on this point: sleep *is* necessary.

What relevance, an insomniac may ask, has all this academic discussion about function to do with the humdrum but nonetheless agonizing problem of the wretch who can't get to sleep? At one time I was inclined to answer "Precious little," though now I'm not so sure. It does seem to me understandable that sleep scientists should have been held back in clinical research into the causes of insomnia because of their inability to answer satisfactorily the basic question what sleep is for.

Yet when that extenuating argument has been raised, it remains disappointing, to say the least, that so little of direct value to insomniacs has come out of the sleep laboratories. Very few of the hundreds of articles in specialist journals on different aspects of sleep have had any connection with the subject. Some indeed appear irrelevant by any criterion. The January 1972 issue of *Sleep Study Abstracts* (which provides a running bibliography on sleep research) reports on the following contributions, among others: "The Dreams of Homosexual and Heterosexual Subjects to the Same Erotic Movie," "Insomnia in Kidney Transplant Patients," "Effects of Early EEG Feedback Training on Sleep Spindle-burst Developments in Kittens" and "An Investigation of Dream

Content among Male Pre-Operative Transsexuals." It may be impertinent for an outsider to say this, but anyone looking at *Sleep Study Abstracts* cannot help but reflect that a good deal of sleep research has been concerned with trivial or eccentric issues. Of course this kind of grumble can be made about any field of scientific research, especially in its early stages; it's hard enough for an insider to know in advance which lines of inquiry are going to prove fruitful and which barren. Yet it is clear that despite the high investment in sleep studies in many parts of the world, clinical research directly aimed to alleviate the miseries of chronic insomnia has up till now been shamefully neglected.

Why should this be? I found an answer of sorts in a paper entitled *Laboratory Studies in Insomnia*, by Allan Rechtschaffen and Lawrence J. Monroe:

> There are several reasons for the lack of active research on insomnia. One seems to be an implicit feeling among investigators that an understanding of insomnia may have to await a more complete understanding of the mechanisms of sleep and wakefulness themselves. Also, it appears, there is an implicit feeling that insomnia has a low priority among the ills that plague us. People do not seem to die of insomnia, and it would be hard to visualize an urgent heart-rending appeal for an American Insomnia Foundation. But it would also be hard to convince a chronic insomniac in his tossing and turning that his disorder is not serious. Furthermore, we really have no good evidence of just how serious insomnia is apart from subjective discomfort. Does it cause personal maladjustment? How seriously does it interfere with productivity? Does it really lower resistance to other diseases? Does it affect longevity itself? There is almost no systematic research on these questions.*

These are not the only questions one might ask. Dr. Wilkinson, working at the Applied Psychology Unit in Cambridge, has offered us, through controlled measurements of performance, a valuable criterion for assessing the quality of

---

*From *Sleep: Physiology and Pathology*, ed. A. Kales (Philadelphia: Lippincott, 1969).

sleep, but we also need to know how to improve that quality, how to get the greatest benefit from a given amount of sleep. The application of these techniques to an individual's sleep requirements would need a lot of extra support from the Medical Research Council.

No one knows to what extent people suffer from insomnia, because there is as yet no agreement as to what insomnia is. It may be a specific disease or, like fever, simply a symptom of other disorders. Because we don't know the extent, we have no idea what it is costing society in terms of poor work or avoidable accidents, or what it is costing individuals in unnecessary suffering. At every turn we meet fundamental questions waiting to be answered. Almost certainly they will continue to wait until greater funds are forthcoming, and funds earmarked specifically for insomniac research. The sleep clinic described on pp. 41 ff. is a hopeful beginning, but we shall need many more sleep clinics if insomnia is to have the attention it deserves.

Rechtschaffen and Monroe say they cannot envisage a succesful appeal for an Insomnia Foundation. I believe they are wrong, and that such an appeal would meet with an enthusiastic response. Yet it is certainly striking that, up till now, there has been no sign of any pressure group to lobby for research support. If insomnia is to be given more priority when it comes to funding research, then chronic insomniacs will need to acquire the courage of their complaints and make their voices heard.

An Insomnia Foundation is the long-term answer. In the meantime, how about an Insomniacs Anonymous? It would surely help if poor sleepers could meet and talk about their difficulties and ways of coping, if they could be available on bad nights at the other end of a telephone or if, as a group in New York have done, they could organize nocturnal bicycle rides through quiet, empty streets? Insomniacs Anonymous may only be a palliative, but at least it would help to ease the desperate isolation of chronic victims.

The Function of Dreaming

BY CHRISTOPHER EVANS

No one really understands what goes on when we dream, but since Freud there have been plenty of theories from which to choose. Dr. Christopher Evans, an experimental psychologist in the Computer Science Division of the British National Physical Laboratory, elaborates on this concept: drawing a parallel between computers and living systems, he sees dreaming as a vital process of the brain for separating useful from useless experiences. But he goes further: to Dr. Evans, the whole purpose of sleep is to allow us to dream. I can see difficulties in this view: if dreaming is all-important, how is it that many individuals whose dream periods are inhibited by tranquilizers show no signs of ill effects and that depressive patients can actually be helped if they are deprived of their dreaming? Nevertheless, Dr. Evans' contribution to the great sleep debate is one of the most imaginative and stimulating that I have come across.

~~~~~~~~~~~~~~~~~~~~~~~~~~~~~~~~~~~~

Thanks to a series of ingenious and incisive experiments in recent years, we are now on the brink of a revolution—a revolution in our thinking about sleep and dreams. These experiments have provoked a theory that may enable us to explain, once and for all, why we sleep, why we dream, and why people need less sleep as they grow older. Because of these experiments, we may also be able to determine whether the psychoanalytic theory of dreams and sleep has any validity. Finally, we may even be in a position to answer that provocative question, Can we ever sleep less—recover part of the one-third of our lives we spend sleeping?

Up to now, theories of sleep and dreams have fallen into three broad groups:

> the common-sense theory;
> the fantastical theory; and
> the psychoanalytic theory.

With the coming of the experimental findings of the past decade, a fourth theory has emerged, one we might call the "functional" theory. Let us take up all four of them in order.

The most common-sense view of sleep is that it is a period of rest for both body and brain after the day's hectic activities. The support for this approach is obvious. First, physical activity clearly slows down during sleep: so, apparently, does mental activity, for sleep—except when "disturbed" by dreams—seems to be a period of mental blankness, when thinking, learning, remembering, and so on, come to a halt and the individual, for all practical purposes, ceases to exist. Second, after a "sound" sleep we rise feeling refreshed, both physically and mentally. "Rest" would seem to be the prime cause. Dreams, by this view, are held to be weird intrusions into the sleep state, breakdowns in the brain's smooth rest cure, and they are to be avoided at all costs if a person is to get "a good night's sleep."

Unfortunately for this pleasingly simple hypothesis, there are some annoyingly contrary facts that have been around in one form or another for some decades and that give the common-sense view a bit of a knock. In the first place, it is simply not true that sleep is essential for bodily rest: the body's tissues are self-restoring and require relatively little inactivity. In fact, they function best when more or less continuously active, and need only brief periods of pause after persistent effort, the sort of pause achieved by an hour or so in an armchair. During sleep, in addition, there are regular periods of muscular movement specifically meant to *prevent* muscular inactivity.

As for the brain's resting, this might be a plausible hypothesis were it not for the interesting data from electroencephalography, data showing that, while there is a significant change in the *nature* of the EEG recordings during sleep (a shift toward the slower, high-amplitude waves), there is no indication whatsoever that there is any *less* activity going on. Both of these are critical objections to the most commonly held view of sleep and dreams.

The popularity of the second theory, the fantastical, has declined somewhat in recent years (it is probably the oldest of the theories), but it is still very widely held, even if in a pseudo-sophisticated form. This theory is really a great set of subtheories, all more or less plausible according to one's upbringing and inclinations, but at root all are manifestations of a single theme: during sleep, the soul or spirit is free to leave the body, and dreams are the soul's adventures during its free roaming. A modern variety of this—and one no less fantastic and no more scientific—is the version beloved by the Victorian psychical researcher and, in more restrained form, by the twentieth-century parapsychologist. Here the mind, during sleep, is in some strange way released from the shackles of the material world, and may either communicate "telepathically" with other uninhibited minds or receive special information about calamities of significance to the sleeper. Hence the portentous dreams of distant deaths and future events that make Myers and Gurney's *Phantasms of the Living* such a spine-tingling book, and that make up the bulk of J. W. Dunne's exercise in precognitive dreams, *An Experiment with Time*.

This theory is difficult to refute, but (personal preferences aside) much hinges, of course, on the general probability of the mind-body duality and of the existence of telepathy. The philosophical complications of the former have long been well-known, while the scientific evidence for the latter, once considerable, now seems to be dwindling rapidly. We will not take this further here, but just suggest that this interesting theory now seems too far out of tune with the world, at least as we know it, to be any longer acceptable.

The most exciting and startling development in our understanding of sleep and dreams—until the very latest developments—has come from the Vienna school of psychoanalysis, and in particular from the tremendous insights of Sigmund Freud. Through the technique of free association and the meticulous analysis of patients' dreams, Freud gradually became aware that dream content reflected (though often in weirdly distorted form) the individual's powerful emotional drives and conflicts. At first a hunch, this was soon built into the form of a theory which declared that dreams represented the pent-up emotional stresses and basic desires that the pressures of social conformity force us to repress or deny. In sleep, with the "social censor" off guard, these repressed but still dynamic forces thrust to the surface as dreams. Hence the great importance attached by psychoanalysts, then and now, to the content of dreams as clues to a person's true personality.

This view of dreaming, with its extensive implications for theories of personality and motivation, and even for religious and moral beliefs, made relatively rapid headway in medico-scientific circles, although taking half a century to arouse more than jocular incredulity among lay people. But anyone who has spent any time at all pondering the content of his own dream life will have little doubt about the validity of much of the psychoanalytic approach.

On the other hand, to all but the thoroughly indoctrinated, the gross deficiencies of the theory as a comprehensive approach will be obvious. To take the most glaring difficulty, what are we to make of those dreams, which we all experience at one time or another, that consist of simple, day-to-day happenings, quite clearly devoid of deep emotional significance? Psychoanalytic theory is well aware of this dangerous loophole, and has postulated a theory that dreams disguise their real meaning through bizarre distortions and cunningly planted red herrings—the disguise being to prevent the startling nature of the repressed material from disturbing the dreamer's sleep and thus awakening him. This ingeniously gets over the criticism, but, alas, it hangs psychoanalytic theory on the hook more firmly than ever; it forces the dream interpreter into ever more desperate searches for deeply significant hidden meanings in totally innocuous dream material. The result has been that a slight air of levity, of the music-hall-joke variety, has surrounded the relationship between the psychoanalyst and his interpretation of dreams.

Nevertheless, despite the drawbacks to the single-minded psychoanalytic theory of dreams, it is the theory that has remained undisputed master of the arena until recently.

In the late 1950's Dr. William Dement and colleagues at the Mount Sinai Hospital in New York began a series of experiments that were to have a more profound effect on the whole topic of sleep and dreams than any previous experimental approach. Of particular interest was the finding that when the subjects were awakened during one of these rapid-eye-movement (REM) periods, they reported that they were—at the time of awakening—experiencing a dream. Surprise number two came when the amount of time devoted to dreaming (as measured by this new behavioural index) was counted up. Young adults, it was found, spent as much as 25 percent of their sleeping time in REM periods, and this percentage was even appreciably greater on certain occasions.

Dr. Dement had been quick to see that the extraordinary amount of time young adults spent dreaming suggested that dreaming had an important function. This possibility might be tested by depriving subjects of the opportunity to dream—by interrupting their REM periods. His experiment revealed that subjects deprived of REM activity for several nights on end seemed to show behavioural and psychological disturbances. A control group, kept awake for an equal amount of time but *not* during REM periods, remained, to all appearances, normal. Psychologists, psychiatrists, and psychoanalysts all over the world pricked up their ears. Perhaps the real purpose of sleep was to allow us to *dream!*

Since then, Dr. Dement's experiment—with modifications—has been repeated in many laboratories, and its principal findings have not been effectively challenged. Subsequent experiments, in fact, strengthened the original idea. For example, it was found that subjects who had been deprived of REM periods for some nights, when finally left to sleep normally, *spent a greater percentage of the sleep period in REM activity than they did under normal conditions.* Enforced reduction in dreaming time led to more dreaming in later sleep sessions.

These findings, which may be some of the most significant in the history of modern psychological research, seem to make it quite clear that sleep is *not* a period of rest or mental blankness, but a period designed to allow some kind of dynamic, and probably vital, process to take place. But what kind of process can this be?

Pondering the function and nature of this process led a colleague, computer expert Ted Newman, and me to propose an analogy between dreaming and one type of computer activity. Let me explain. The more complex living brains seem to contain two repositories of memory—one short-term and the other more permanent. This is the "dual-memory-system" hypothesis. According to this hypothesis, events a person has experienced are first held in some labile system that has a high storage capacity but a restricted life. Then these events are accepted or rejected for long-term storage according to a built-in set of criteria. Events that pass the "usefulness" test are then transferred to the permanent store. "Rejects"—redundant material, erroneous actions—are totally disposed of, perhaps by the discharge of some kind of electrical circuit.

Now, for some time I had been trying to relate dreaming to the dual-memory-system hypothesis. I had made no effort to work out the theory in detail, but it did seem to me that dreaming might correspond to the discharge of the short-term memory store. Dreaming might, in other words, be a way of rejecting useless memories. And when a dream is interrupted by the sleeper's awakening, it seemed to me, this would cause the dream to be "experienced" and perhaps transferred to the permanent memory store. For this to be true, some form of scanning of the material held in the short-term store—a selection and classification procedure—must be taking place when a person dreams. As it stood, the theory, if one can call it that, was little better than a slightly more up-to-date version of the "dreams as mental defecation" idea, which is quite venerable in one form or another. An important insight, however, came after Newman and I had been discussing certain activities of advanced and complex computers.

Computers perform a variety of complex tasks according to a set of programs —instructions to the machine to use its analytic equipment in a certain way. As computers develop in size and complexity, and as the range of tasks for which they are equipped increases, it becomes gradually more important for the programs to be regularly revised and reclassified—in order to bring the computer up-to-date. Take computers that control the wage and salary system for a large firm. As wages increase, taxes change and the size of the payroll varies. So the computer's programs must constantly be altered. Now, as things stand with today's relatively simple-minded computers, this program clearance may be done by a technician. He takes the computer "off-line" (uncouples it from the task it is controlling), then runs the programs through and makes modifications where necessary. In order to perform this set of operations, it is imperative that the computer be "off-line." Otherwise, the experimental or modified programs will do the job they were intended to do *as they are being run through.*

So, if there is an error in the program, we would get sets of peculiar pay checks coming up at the wrong time, or worse, if the computer were controlling operations in some form of chemical factory, disastrous explosions might result.

Our brain-computer analogy states that the purpose of sleep is to take a man's brain "off-line"—to prepare for revising and clearing the brain's programs in the light of recent events and experiences. Dreaming, by this analogy, is the *running through of the programs and their reclassifications*. Yet we normally are not aware of this clearance of experiences. Only when the process is interrupted, because of some external or internal disturbance of the sleeper, will consciousness interact with the clearance activity, *and what we popularly call a dream* be experienced. A dream is thus either a useful or a useless experience that is being classified.

In short, sleep is a process *intended* to allow us to dream, and to dream without interruption from the external world (which might muddle up existing programs) and without the program-clearance operation interacting with the world in a positive fashion (we are not, unfortunately, completely "off-line" when we sleep-talk or sleepwalk).

The content of most dreams, incidentally, is probably trivial, since most of our experiences are of the useless variety. At first thought, this seems to conflict with one's own subjective impressions. The apparent significance of much of our dreaming can be understood, however, when we remember that we are talking about *interrupted* dreams in this context, and that it is dreams with great *effect*, and provoking autonomic bodily reactions, that are most likely to wake us up. The vast bulk of undisturbed dreaming, in fact, will probably consist of very drab, routine material—the bread-and-butter experiences of the previous day being fitted into the program system. Occasionally we become aware of this boring rubbish when a fever brings fitful sleep. Then we see dreams for what they really are: endless sessions of counting; reading nonsense; attempts to solve weird problems; driving vast distances; and so on. To slightly misquote an acknowledged expert on the topic, this is really "the stuff of dreams," and we should be very glad that we normally sleep through it all.

What might be the effect of interfering persistently with this memory-clearing activity? Computers whose programs are not modified regularly get progressively less and less efficient at their jobs, and programs could become badly muddled if classification processes broke down. Humans, when deprived of sleep, and therefore of dreaming, become muddled and confused, and soon find all but the simplest of tasks difficult. In due course, there may be psychotic episodes, and hallucinations (emergency waking dreams?) may appear.

We may be a long way from computers hallucinating, but one can easily imagine that some form of automatic program-clearance system might usefully be built into the very complex and comprehensive computers of the not too distant future. Those of us who are of a fanciful turn of mind might like to call *this* dreaming.

Dr. Dement's exciting and original experiments, in addition to provoking this "functional" theory of sleep and dreams, also oblige us to change our view of that third portion of our lives that we had considered to be empty and lost. Thus, a recent science-fiction novel, and more than one short story, has had as its theme the possibility of reclaiming the sleeping hours. This kind of speculation no longer makes sense now, and suggests that an important change in attitude may be necessary. One obvious example comes to mind. If the program-clearance analogy is a good one, then we should expect significant differences in sleep (dream) requirements with age. *New* material affects existing programs the most, and in youth, when our sensory-gathering equipment is at the peak of its efficiency and our ability to learn is the greatest, we will therefore require the most sleep. With old age, and its obvious concomitants, sleep requirements should drastically fall off. Old people, then, should be taught to accept their lack of need for sleep and, where possible, learn to enjoy the hours they have gradually regained.

A second change of attitude that may be necessary concerns our use of drugs. The level of sleep needed for "good dreaming" to take place might be quite precise, and one can imagine that certain drugs might well depress the individual *below* this level. (Recent experiments by Jouvet in France indicate that the REM phase *is* inhibited by barbiturates.) Conversely, hallucinogenic drugs, including LSD in its various forms, might produce their effects by activating the dream mechanism at unsuitable times—in particular when the brain is not "off-line." The dangers of permanent interference with the dreaming process could be great, and the hallucinogens might be fearfully risky to play with.

Finally, what are we now to think of psychoanalytic theories of dreams? Curiously, in an important way, it seems to me that psychoanalytic theory is helped rather than hindered—because the analyst is relieved of the need to observe or uncover significance in every remembered dream. Dreams of emotional and psychoanalytic importance will, of course, still occur, their frequency depending on the role that their subject matter plays in the patient's waking life. They will be just as revealing to dream analysis. The good analyst, however, will now need to learn to distinguish between the genuinely significant and the genuinely trivial in the individual's dream life.

The Sleep Clinic

BY MAGGIE SCARF

Useful information about insomnia is slowly, but oh so slowly, percolating through to the general medical practitioner. One of the more hopeful developments in recent years has been the advent of sleep clinics offering specialist diagnosis and help to those suffering from sleep disorders. Maggie Scarf here describes one of the only three such clinics in the United States. Russia, Germany, Austria, France and Israel have sleep clinics, but there are none as yet in Britain. The time may well be coming, however, when every self-respecting major hospital will require its own sleep department as it already has its clinic for, say, orthopedics or gynecology.

~~~~~~~~~~~~~~~~~~~~~~~~

It was 11:15 P.M. Most of the electrodes had already been pasted into place.

One was behind each of the patient's ears and one above each eye; two were on her chin and three on her forehead—these five were for measuring muscular tension. There was also a single electrode to the right of her nostrils, for measuring the rate of breathing. Now Dr. Peter Hauri, director of the Dartmouth Sleep Laboratory at Hanover, New Hampshire, was positioning two more electrodes on the very top of the patient's head, just over the parietal lobes of the brain; these were for picking up and recording her brain waves. "You know," said the woman apprehensively, "I have an awful time getting to sleep ordinarily. I don't see how I'm ever going to sleep with all these wires coming out of my head."

"Oh, don't worry about trying too hard to sleep," Dr. Hauri said cheerfully. "You'll get off eventually; everybody does. *Everybody* sleeps in my lab." He placed an electrode under the patient's armpit and anchored it firmly with a strip of translucent tape; this one was for monitoring body temperature. A final electrode went on the middle of her back—for measuring heart rate. "O.K.," he said, "now you're all ready for sleep."

Lifting the trail of wires like a bridal train, Dr. Hauri walked behind her, directing her out and into the hallway, then into the small, comfortable-looking sleeping room next door. There, helping her as she settled herself in the bed, he assured her that he would be available, via the intercom system, throughout the night. He would come to her immediately should she summon him. As he talked, he was carefully plugging the wires into jacks in a small panel just over the bed.

"Doctor, that big machine in your laboratory—I guess these wires here must connect up with it. And I was wondering—if one of the fuses shorted out or something like that, the electricity—it couldn't go into my head, could it?" She laughed slightly, as if embarrassed.

"You're not the only person who's been worried about that," he replied, his German-accented voice courteous and full of sympathy. "But I assure you that it is really completely safe. Hundreds of sleep subjects have been tested on these machines and no one—*not one single person*—has ever been harmed in even the slightest way."

Back in the laboratory, Dr. Hauri began checking the polygraph recordings as they started to emerge from the electroencephalograph, or brain-wave recording machine. He was also monitoring heart-rate variability, body temperature, breathing rate and muscle tension as well. The patient was, at the moment, still tossing and turning; the needles tracing muscular tension were fluctuating wildly.

As he began to calibrate several of the dials, Dr. Hauri told me something about this woman's sleep history. She had had severe and chronic insomnia for thirty years. Now in her early fifties, she managed only about three hours of sleep a night—and only with the aid of heavy dosages of pills.

"At least," said Dr. Hauri, "she *thinks* the sleeping drug is the only thing that will get her any respite at all. The fact is, however, that if the medication has any effect in inducing sleep in this patient, it is at this point a purely psychological one. For, as has been shown in sleep study after sleep study, the hypnotics—I mean all sleeping pills—become ineffective after two or three, or at the very outside, four weeks of steady use. After that period of time, they simply don't work.

"You know, there is a very familiar pattern to all this, we see it time after time. An individual starts out by taking one of these sleep medications; he takes a single pill at night, and that's just fine. Then, perhaps after a week or two, he needs a couple of those pills to get the same results. And then, after a while, that doesn't have the same effect either—but he keeps on with the pills because, without them, he sleeps even worse. Well, what has happened in this situation is really quite commonplace: the person is not being helped by the pills at all any more; meanwhile, he's gotten himself hooked on the drug.

"I'm not saying that the sleeping pills won't continue to have a psychological effect long after they've ceased to have a physiological one. In other words, the individual may, because he *believes* the drug is putting him to sleep, actually be able to relax enough so that he can doze off . . . But the pill itself isn't doing a thing. On the contrary, the pills are most probably going to disturb the pattern of his sleep, and his sleep is certainly going to be far more rotten because he's taken them."

As he spoke to me Dr. Hauri was keeping an eye on the lines of data steadily being recorded on the machine. He pointed out the one denoting the patient's muscle tension: it had changed dramatically, and now looked smaller and as evenly drawn as a design. The patient's heart rate was steady, her breathing deep and uniform. The brain waves were in the alpha—"awake but resting" —phase. If her sleep pattern ran true to her descriptions of it, she would now, Dr. Hauri told me, lie awake for several hours doing something which she called "fidgeting." Then, toward two or three in the morning, she would resort to two capsules of her sleep medication. After that she would doze off for perhaps three to three-and-a-half hours, then lie awake again. "One thing that we do see all the time with insomniacs is that they stay in bed without being asleep much more than other people do—much too long. They are there for hours before falling asleep; and the same thing happens when they awake in the morning as well."

Much to my surprise, however, before even so much as an hour passed, the patient began the slow descent into sleep. Muscular tension had diminished again; the "design" looked even more regular, the waves lower in amplitude. Her brain-wave pattern was showing the mixed-frequency, "half-awake, half-asleep," somewhat slower configuration of Stage I, the lightest phase of sleep. A normal sleeper would have stayed at this level for no more than a few minutes. But in the patient's case it persisted for over half an hour.

Then she shuttled downward into Stage II. Some researchers consider Stage II no more than the prelude, the gateway, to the more profound—the restorative, recuperative—phases of sleep represented by stages III or IV. These deeper stages are characterized by the appearance of delta waves on the EEG recording: large, slow, rolling waves that are sometimes about five times the amplitude of the waking alpha rhythm. Delta waves have a satisfying appearance: they look like brain waves of deep slumber *ought* to look—lazy and easy and wide. The only real differentiation between stages III and IV is that recordings made during the latter stage show a higher percentage of delta waves.

In this particular instance, however, the patient was unlikely to exhibit any of the deep-sleep pattern at all. "The sleeping pills have, most likely, knocked out all of her delta sleep," said Dr. Hauri. "And even though she hasn't had the pills so far this evening, the fact that she's been on them so long will mean that this kind of sleep is being pretty much obliterated."

In fact, she never did descend into the lower stages of healthy slumber, as a normal sleeper would have done. An individual with no sleep pathology would have gone downward to the stage III and IV levels, then returned slowly upward, to enter into a first REM—or "rapid eye movement" period, when the eyeballs dart vigorously under closed eyelids—some ninety minutes after the onset of sleep. This patient, however, went directly from stage II sleep into a lengthy REM period. Her elevated heart rate, irregular breathing and "wakeful" brain-wave pattern continued for almost half an hour. Then, abruptly, she woke up.

Nocturnal awakenings, Dr. Hauri told me, are nothing out of the ordinary even for normal sleepers; adults generally awaken some three to five times during a healthy night's sleep. Most people, however, return to sleep at once and retain no memory of these brief awakenings. The individual with a sleep disorder, on the other hand, tends to wake up more frequently and once awake, finds getting back to sleep either difficult or impossible.

This was indeed what happened. The patient lay in her bed, tossing and "fidgeting" until close to three in the morning; then she took two sleeping capsules. Shortly afterward, she fell into a long Stage I sleep, and then spent a briefer time in Stage II. This time she returned to Stage I without having any REM period at all. The medication, now metabolizing through her system, was suppressing the dream phase of normal sleep. All sleeping pills, including even the mild over-the-counter antihistamines, affect REM sleep profoundly; so do anti-anxiety drugs such as tranquilizers, and so do alcohol and amphetamines. Antidepressant drugs also act to inhibit or erase dreaming sleep.

One fascinating clue which did emerge from the night's sleep-recording session was the curious fact that the patient believed she had not slept until she took her pills at 3 A.M. In an interview with Dr. Hauri the following morning, she said that up until three o'clock she had lain awake "fidgeting." And yet, according to objective standards—the recorded EEG readings—she had actually fallen asleep within an hour of retiring.

"Her own subjective experience is that she didn't sleep until she took the pills," Dr. Hauri told me after he had spoken with her. "And this makes me suspect that she may be, in part, suffering from a condition called 'pseudo insomnia'—she's actually sleeping, but dreaming that she's awake. I've had such cases before: the worst was a student here at Dartmouth who used to get a full eight hours' sleep every night, but spent all his REM periods dreaming that he was awake. He was exhausted by morning."

As he talked, Dr. Hauri was beginning to write out instructions for the sleep technician who would be monitoring the same patient the following night. He planned to have the assistant speak to the woman during the time of night when the EEG readings indicated that she was asleep, although she believed herself to be awake. "I'll have the technician simply *talk* to *her*, ask her if she thinks she's sleeping or not. And then, when we see what she answers, we'll know better what has been going on in her mind.

"We won't, by the way," he added, "come up with any magical solutions; not in the 'Eureka!' sense of the word. What we will come up with is, very likely, a reasonable hypothesis about what might be causing the sleep disturbance . . . I mean, whether it is neurological in origin, or secondary to some medical or psychological problem, or something else. And this educated guess will be followed by a list of several recommendations about what that person then might do. Usually—in about 75 to 80 percent of our cases—one of these recommendations will work well, and we'll get a cure: the person will be able to sleep much better."

Informal estimates indicate that about 20 million Americans probably suffer from some form of sleep disturbance. A Department of Health, Education and Welfare report, covering the years 1952–1963 stated that while sales of all drugs had increased 6.5 percent during this period, retail sales of hypnotics and tranquilizers had increased 535 percent. One can only imagine what the rise may have been in the decade just past—no hard statistics are available. And yet, despite the fact that a large untreated "sleep-patient" population patently does exist, there are only three formal sleep clinics—laboratories whose main function is to treat patients rather than to carry out sleep experiments (although some laboratories primarily oriented toward research do occasionally take a few private patients)—in the entire nation. One is, of course, the Dartmouth Laboratory. Another is located at Hershey, Pennsylvania. The third, and by far the largest, is in California at the Stanford University School of Medicine complex.

The Dartmouth Sleep Laboratory, although part of the Dartmouth-Hitchcock Medical Center, is very small. It is the Swiss-born Peter Hauri's own baby. A clinical psychologist with a Ph.D. from the University of Chicago, Dr. Hauri is assisted by a group of trained sleep technicians; he also works in close consultation with the varied medical specialists and psychiatric experts connected with the Dartmouth-Hitchcock Center.

If sleep clinics are few in number, and all fairly new, it is because the entire field of sleep research has just begun to consolidate—and to try to apply—what has been a virtual explosion of new information. Obviously, if sleep specialists were to offer counseling on specific disorders, they needed to have some basic understanding of the normal patterns of human sleep—otherwise, what was the standard against which they could make comparisons? How could one help a person with a problem unless one were fully aware of what constituted a normal night's sleep?

Such fundamental information has become available only recently. Indeed, more has been learned about sleep in the past decade and a half than during the rest of human history. Studies have demonstrated that normal sleepers, within roughly similar age ranges, will show a remarkable consistency in the course and pattern of their sleep. Healthy sleepers are pretty much alike. For the sleep clinician it is the particular infrastructure, the form and shape of a patient's sleep (as it is recorded by sophisticated laboratory instrumentation) that is far more important than the length of that sleep. Indeed, analysis of the sleep of individuals with very long or short sleeping periods will sometimes reassure the patient with a "sleep problem" that there is, in fact, no problem at all.

"We had a seventy-year-old woman in here recently," remarked Dr. Hauri, "whose husband sent her because he thought she had a sleep disorder; she only slept four hours a night. She told me that she hadn't ever slept much more than four hours a night in her whole life—she thought it was peculiar too.

"Well, we tested her in the laboratory, and there was nothing at all wrong. What she did have was a remarkably efficient sleep. She went very quickly into deep delta slumber, the stage three and four phases. And then, after about an hour-and-a-half of that, up she came: she went directly into a little REM dream period. After that, back down she went, came out once more; then it was all over. And if she didn't have more than a tiny bit of the stage one or stage two intermediate stuff, it was because she didn't actually need more than the four hours of sleep. She was as sound as a bell."

Another patient, a physics professor in his early fifties, came to the sleep laboratory with the reverse problem: he needed fourteen hours of sleep a night. "We had him spend two nights here in the clinic, and we didn't find any disorder in his sleeping at all," says Dr. Hauri. "His pattern was perfectly normal, and it was right for him. He simply *had* to have that fourteen hours.

If he only got twelve hours of sleep, he was exhausted the whole next day."

Sleep disturbances fall into one of three broad categories: problems relating to too little sleep (insomnia), to too much sleep (hypersomnia), and another, more or less wastebasket category which includes all the other disorders (dyssomnia). Included in this last group are such things as persistent nightmares, sleepwalking or sleeptalking.

Walking or talking in one's sleep are usually not related, as is commonly believed, to the "acting out" of the sleeper's dreams. Actually, it would be impossible for an individual to move around or to communicate during the REM, or dream phase, of sleeping. Despite the fact that the sleeper's body is in a physiological state comparable to fright or excitement in waking, and the brain is hyperalert, the sleeper's body musculature is flaccid. Indeed, many postural muscles are paralyzed during this episode of sleep. Some sleep scientists believe that our brains are behaving as if awake during REM, and giving commands to our muscles as usual, but that our bodies cannot respond to these messages, having become temporarily limp.

Although patients with every kind of sleep complaint turn up at the Dartmouth Clinic, the largest group Dr. Hauri sees are those with problems of insomnia. Among the chronic insomniacs, there are distinct subgroups. "We differentiate," Dr. Hauri says, "between the person with a sleep-onset problem, and the guy who *can* get to sleep but has frequent awakenings during the night, and the person who does get to sleep all right, but then snaps wide awake in the early morning hours. This last pattern is, we find, often not primarily a sleep problem; it is frequently secondary to depression. You clear up the depression, and the sleep disturbance disappears."

In treating the three different kinds of insomniacs, Dr. Hauri says, his greatest successes are with the first group, the ones who have chronic difficulties getting to sleep.

"There might be one of a hundred things wrong with a person who can't fall asleep," Dr. Hauri says. "An individual might have some difficulty in metabolizing the serotonin in his brain. Serotonin is the "sleep juice," the brain chemical which is believed to be related to sleep. Or perhaps the patient suffers from some chemical difficulty in making the serotonin out of tryptophane, a precursor to serotonin; tryptophane is in foods like milk, cheese and meat. The tryptophane goes from the food into the blood, and then to the brain, where it's converted into serotonin. You know how you sometimes feel very groggy after a heavy meal? That's because you have, in a sense, eaten a sleeping pill. There's about a gram of tryptophane in an ordinary-sized steak; and that's enough to make a person quite drowsy."

This extraordinary piece of information prompted me to confess, on the spot, that every night just before going to bed I myself have a cup of hot milk, usually mixed with Ovaltine. He laughed: "Ovaltine has, in fact, been shown to be helpful in inducing sleep. A 1937 study, done by Nathaniel Kleitman, demonstrated this." Another study, Dr. Hauri told me, which was more recent but equally respectable, demonstrated that the bedtime milk-and-cereal drink called Horlick's was also a "natural" hypnotic. "Warm milk at night is good, too, and not only because it smells like mother, but because there is tryptophane in the stuff. But the effects of these things are not, of course, all that strong. If we have somebody who is a real insomniac, neither of these warm-milk drinks is going to overcome that."

Treatment, for two patients presenting themselves at the sleep clinic with seemingly identical problems—for instance, an inability to fall asleep—may be radically different. This is because the therapy a person receives will always depend on an analysis of his sleeping pattern, and the clues that turn up regarding the possible causes of the disorder. The same kind of symptom—for example, sleep-onset disturbance—may stem from any one of a variety of conditions. The problem may be neurological in origin, and related to degeneration of nerve cells deep in the brain. Or it may be genetic, or may be caused by myoclonic seizures—those strange muscular jerks that most of us have experienced while falling asleep—which go on and on, waking the individual every time he is about to fall asleep. Or the disorder may be secondary to some organic difficulty—a persistent low-grade headache or minor pain which can be pushed from awareness during the day's activity, but which becomes more insistent during the stillness of the night. Or the problem may be psychological in origin.

Sometimes a sleep disturbance is even related to a difficulty long since worked through and solved. "This is something which we call a 'functionally autonomous' onset problem," says Dr. Hauri. "It's a situation in which there was, at one time, a reason why a person couldn't sleep. Maybe the reason was even medical; most likely, it was psychological. And so, for a period of time— maybe a month, maybe more—the individual was not able to fall asleep easily. After that, the person got himself into a cycle where he hated the night because he dreaded not being able to sleep, but he couldn't sleep because that dread got him too tensed up. In this kind of case the individual has, somewhere along the line, become conditioned to his bedtime environment. The pillow, the bed, the lamp, etc., are not cues for drowsiness but for increased alertness and arousal. And so he starts tossing and turning."

Even though the initial problem which originally caused such a person to lose sleep may be solved—indeed, may have been solved twenty years earlier—he is left with the sleep disturbance which began at that time. These people often sleep much better in very dissimilar kinds of environments; not infrequently, they go right off to sleep in the laboratory.

Patients treated for this kind of sleep-onset disorder may follow a regime (first developed by psychologist Richard R. Bootzin) that attempts to recondition them to the bedtime stimuli that have been serving as signals for tension and wakefulness. The patient is told that if he is not sleeping when he is in bed, then he is misusing the bed. The bed is only for sleeping. And he is forbidden to lie in it, tossing and turning—for that, as he is informed in no uncertain terms, is counterproductive.

The patient is enjoined not to lie in bed awake for more than about ten minutes; if he has not fallen asleep within this period, he must get up and leave the room. He is to do all his worrying, all his thinking about his shortcomings, away from the bedroom situation.

If after an hour, three hours (or sometimes twelve hours or more), the patient feels ready to sleep, he may return to the bed, hit the pillow and fall asleep. If, however, he fails to do so in the five to ten minutes allotted, he has to get up and go out again—he is misusing the bed. He must follow this regimen even if it means staying up throughout the entire night. There is one final admonition for the patient: he must not sleep late, even if he manages to fall asleep a mere five minutes before the time he should be awakening for the next day.

"On the first night of this treatment the patient usually won't sleep at all; he'll feel miserable the whole day after. But the following night, being tired, he'll get off to sleep somewhere about three or four in the morning. The night

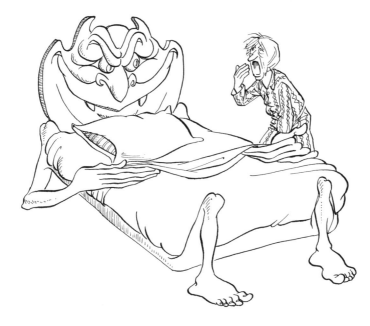

after that he stays awake for something like three hours. The next night, it might be two. And then the individual gets happy, because he sees that it's going to work. Within about two to three weeks, many chronic insomniacs can be retrained in this way so that they can just hit the pillow and fall asleep.

"But it does," Dr. Hauri acknowledges, "take a good deal of fortitude: at five A.M., say, when a person still isn't sleeping, and he knows there's a full day's work ahead of him. And once again he has to get out of that bed because he is misusing it. Most often a patient will need someone behind him, some sleep or behavioral therapist, to hold his hand and tell him that he's doing fine and that things are sure to get better."

Serotonin is the neurochemical in the brain which is related, it appears, not only to falling asleep but to that profound delta sleep of the Stage IV phase. Another chemical in the brain, norepinephrine, is believed to mediate the REM, or dreaming phases, of our sleep. Any substance which affects delicate brain chemistry—most specifically, the norepinephrine and serotonin levels—will influence both our sleeping and dreaming patterns. Unfortunately, all known sleeping drugs *do* affect brain neurochemicals, and all distort or suppress one phase or another of normal sleep.

"I am not," Dr. Hauri assured me, "against sleeping pills for the guy or the woman with an occasional sleep problem. We all, in the course of events, get into some situation or another where we cannot sleep at night; I do too. The main thing is not to exaggerate the importance of losing a night's sleep. It might make a person *feel* bad, but as a number of studies have shown, it will have practically no effect upon his objective efficiency. It would take three or four nights of no sleep at all before his ability to perform actually went down.

"But if an individual is getting himself all uptight and into some sort of a bind about his inability to sleep; and if this should continue for a few nights running, then he might be moving into a vicious cycle—that 'functionally autonomous' sleep-onset problem. So for myself, if I start getting miserable, I'll take a sleeping pill and that will knock me out. I know, however, that the pill-induced sleep will be lousy, because hypnotic drugs suppress the dreaming phase of sleep. And then, the following night, I would expect something which is called the 'REM rebound': that is, in that next sleep period I'd be making up for the dreams that were suppressed the night before."

The "dream rebound" is what makes it so hard for people who are hooked on sleeping drugs to get off them. "The first night they try to make it without the pills they get this horrible sleep—it's virtually all REM, and full of anxiety dreams and nightmares," explained Dr. Hauri. "That's why you can't take people off the sleeping drugs 'cold turkey'; REM rebound hits them, and they become terrified." Withdrawal from the chronic use of sleep medications must always, he cautions, be done very gradually—and if at all possible, under the supervision of a doctor. If a habitual user suddenly ceases taking his sleeping pills, he may suffer such serious effects as convulsions, delirium, hallucinations, hypertension.

"To get a patient off drugs, I try to give him something else. Something like progressive relaxation exercises that he can do by himself, to relax his body muscles—and which will keep him from feeling so utterly helpless. Or I may start him out with some form of biofeedback: we've been trying that out recently, with good success. Biofeedback involves, very simply, taking some parameter of the patient's body—his brain waves or his muscle tension, something not usually under his control—and measuring those brain waves or the tension in those muscles, and then displaying that measure to the person himself. When a patient can observe, say, his muscle tension, he can begin to learn what it is that he unconsciously does that tends to increase or decrease it. In this way he can eventually learn to control it."

The same relaxed state which is related to decreased muscle tension is associated with "letting go," to decathexis from the environment—to falling asleep. When a person has managed to get himself hooked on sleeping medications, he has to start out by becoming adept either at the relaxation exercises, or at some sort of biofeedback. Only then can he begin cutting down on the pills.

"We literally do just that," Dr. Hauri explained, "cut off pieces of the pill. We chisel off a very little bit at a time. Meanwhile, we are doing our best to control the REM rebound, to reintroduce the dreaming sleep in such a way that it won't get him too anxious or upset."

That long history of sleeping-drug involvement was going to be a major stumbling block in treatment of the woman patient whose sleep Dr. Hauri had monitored last night; that case would be, he said, "a toughie." She was to sleep in the laboratory for another two nights; in the meanwhile, she was undergoing extensive psychological and medical testing. "Our work here is really a sophisticated diagnostic process, which can often reveal quite a lot about the specific factors contributing to a person's sleep problem," Dr. Hauri said.

If, for example, the disorder were related to neurological difficulties, treatment—with appropriate drugs—would be worked out in close consultation with a neurologist. Or if the insomnia appeared to stem from an imbalance of brain chemicals such as serotonin and norepinephrine, drugs that act to inhibit destruction of these substances might be recommended. If the problem seemed connected to some minor medical disorder, careful attention to the medical condition itself would be warranted. Or, if a sleep problem seemed to be caused by a depression which was psychological in origin, a regime of psychotherapy would be prescribed.

Treatments are, obviously, as varied as the sleep disorders themselves are. The best that one can say about "cures" in the sleep clinic is that they appear to be roughly similar to "cures" in medical and psychiatric practice: a few people get dramatically better, most are helped somewhat (and therefore feel and sleep better), and a percentage are not helped in the slightest. These latter patients, according to Dr. Hauri, comprise some 25 percent of his practice: "But many are still not sorry they came. Very often they arrive here believing they've got a condition far more serious than they actually have. And so they do find some comfort in knowing something more specific about what's really going on."

Because so many of the substances which depress REM sleep—like alcohol, tranquilizers and sleeping pills—are in common use, many sleep scientists and clinicians have puzzled over just why we seem to need the REM phase of sleep so urgently. What necessitates that striving to recoup lost dreaming time? During the first spate of dream research in the nineteen-fifties, some experiments carried out by Dr. William Dement (now director of the sleep clinic at the Stanford Medical Center) suggested that dreams, in some inexplicable way, served to maintain the individual's psychological equilibrium—and that loss of dreaming time led to personality disturbances. This is not, it now appears, invariably the case: for example, people suffering from psychological depressions often seem to do better without their REM sleep. And many individuals seem to function adequately over extended periods of time, even though tranquilizers and/or antidepressant medications are suppressing all or much of their REM sleep.

One current theory about REM sleep is that it may be related to the integration of new information into the mass of old information already stored in the brain. This notion seems to have been borne out by a number of recent studies, both with animals and human subjects. Another function of REM sleep appears to be the regulation of some generalized sort of impulse-control mechanism. This might explain why subjects in the Dement study—as well as people taking part in later dream-deprivation experiments—showed increased irritability and aggressiveness. Sometimes they experienced weight gains resulting from a sudden inability to control food intake. The notion that REM sleep is somehow related to impulse control might also explain why depressives often appear to do better without it. The depressed individual frequently has problems connected to harsh overcontrol of his instinctual urges, thoughts and feelings.

Although these theories have done much to explain the function of REM sleep, the need for sleep itself seems puzzling. Why do people and animals sleep at all? Why is sleeping any different, for example, from simply closing one's eyes and resting?

"There is actually a great controversy going on at this moment among sleep scientists about this very problem," said Dr. Hauri when I asked him. "The fact is that nobody has been able to prove that anything basic happens during sleeping, anything which is that different from what happens when we merely lie down and relax. From a strictly neurological and physiological viewpoint, there is no objective proof that any restorative or recuperative processes get under way. And yet we all know, subjectively, that sleep makes us feel better —that we feel refreshed by a good night's sleep, and feel miserable when we're sleepless."

At the present time, there appear to be two opposing theoretical camps among sleep researchers. One group believes that restorative physiological processes get under way during sleep—that there is resynthesis of brain tissue, for example. The other side maintains that our need for sleep is no more than a behavioral adaptation—that the recurrent state of inertia and unresponsiveness which we call sleep has been programmed into us specifically because it promotes survival. They argue that if we take our own species as an example, then it is clear that early man would have been ill-adapted to protecting himself while foraging for food during the dark hours of the night. If he had attempted to function during the darkness, he would have wasted energy uselessly and exposed himself to danger from night predators as well. Therefore, goes the theory, it was necessary for our early ancestors *not* to respond during certain hours of darkness. Sleep is, in this view, essentially a behavior-control mechanism. Dr. Wilse Webb of the University of Florida, the most eloquent spokesman for this theory, points out that the various sleeping patterns of different animal species do not seem to be linked to physiological processes such as the need to synthesize brain protein. There do seem to be, however, curious ties between the sleep and the safety needs of a species. Predators sleep much more than prey; they can afford to relax. The hare and the gazelle sleep little and lightly; the lion may spend up to sixteen hours a day in deep and heavy sleep.

"And yet," I protested to Hauri, "we all make so many distinctions between the qualities of our sleep—whether it's been good or bad, or light or heavy, or too short or long or full of dreams. We all feel so refreshed after a good night, and so destroyed after a night of wakefulness. It seems almost ridiculous to think that, possibly, nothing restorative is going on—that, from a physiological point of view, nothing at all may be happening."

"I know," he said. "It goes against all our common sense. And I, personally, don't believe it myself. But if you asked me to disprove that theory—to offer one shred of evidence to the contrary—I couldn't possibly do it."

"Isn't there some minimum amount of sleep that is necessary simply from the point of view of survival?"

Dr. Hauri shook his head. "There are two cases in the literature—well-documented—of people who just don't sleep at all. One is an Italian farmer; the other is a guy from Australia. These people have been tested in sleep labs, and it is true: they don't sleep. Now, if you compare sleeping to something like fluid intake, you see that there is a real difference—there is a minimum amount of liquid that is necessary for life; without it, a person will dry up and die. But there are individuals who can, apparently, make do without any sleep whatsoever. And they survive."

Electrosleep

BY GAY GAER LUCE AND JULIUS SEGAL

Except for drugs, conventional medicine has had precious little to offer the insomniac. Is it possible that unconventional medicine has solutions worth examining?

Hypnosis, despite its association with show biz and quackery, has for many years been used to alleviate insomnia. Acupuncture is another method of treatment at last winning some kind of general acceptance in the West, and insomnia is among the innumerable complaints it claims to relieve. For the purposes of this book, I consulted eight books on acupuncture to try to discover in exactly what way it helped sleep problems, but was left none the wiser. Acupuncture is a very arcane science! But one prominent acupuncturist I talked to told me that the treatment he offered insomniacs—that is, the precise spots in which he placed his needles—depended on his personal diagnosis of the patient. This in no way discredits acupuncture, which I believe will teach us a great deal when we have time to listen; but it does make it more difficult to explain clearly what happens —let alone why.

A new kind of therapy which is gaining quite rapid ground in medical circles is biofeedback. The central idea behind this technique is the discovery that many biological functions, hitherto believed to be involuntary, can in fact be brought under control. Just as a child learns to direct his arm movements through observation, so biofeedback devices, by "feeding back" a signal to the user, can instruct him as to what is going on in a particular function, and help him to modify it at will. The instruments—small but complicated electronic machines —do not change the user, so it is claimed, but simply allow him to understand and change himself.

Two particular biofeedback devices—the Relaxometer and the Alpha Sensor* —may be helpful to insomniacs. The Relaxometer works through electrodes attached to your fingertips, and helps you to acquire and maintain a state of physical relaxation. While you are relaxed, the machine gives off a low purr; as soon as you tense up, it changes its tone to an unpleasant whine, which gradually diminishes to a low growl and then once again to a purr as you slowly regain your equanimity. This instrument is said to be particularly useful in cases of chronic anxiety and simple phobias, though it is also recommended to busy harassed people who know they need to relax but find it much easier when they have a tone to guide them. The man who markets the Relaxometer in Britain told me that he regularly used his own set for about ten minutes before going to bed if he was at all in a tensed-up condition.

The Relaxometer works on the body. The Alpha Sensor, in contrast, deals with

---

*These are trade names of products marketed both in the United States and in Britain. Manufacturing biofeedback instruments is a growing industry, and there are a number of similar devices available under different names.

the state of the mind, and its electrodes are placed on the scalp. As its name suggests, it is concerned with the alpha rhythms given off by the brain in the pleasantly relaxed stage immediately preceding the onset of sleep. While your brain is registering waves in the frequency range of 8–13 cycles per second, the machine gives off a bleep through its loudspeaker. If the waves move out of this range in either direction, the bleep stops. Through practice, you can learn to empty your mind, for thinking, feeling or using any of your five senses will interfere with alpha production. Zen monks, experienced yogis and transcendental meditators are all said to register a high level of alpha activity when in a state of trance. So the Alpha Sensor may be considered as a kind of technique for controlling consciousness, though the brochure I examined said disarmingly: "There is probably more to the experienced meditator's trance than just strong alpha waves, but they are definitely a part of it."

Using the Alpha Sensor can be an end in itself—an alpha trip may be as relaxing and satisfying and a good deal less dangerous than a trip on drugs— but it obviously can have therapeutic value, too, in calming hyperactive children, for instance, or in helping patients with chronic anxiety conditions. Increasingly hospitals are acquiring these machines for clinical use. And it is also used, though perhaps less than the Relaxometer, by individuals to help them with their personal sleep problems.

As will be evident from the chapter on "Gadgets and Gimmicks, Fads and Fancies" in Part Three, I am somewhat prejudiced on the subject of mechanical sleep devices. There is something noxious, I feel, about courting a natural process like sleep with the products of a technological society as there is in interfering with sleep by means of drugs. But I am convinced that biofeedback can be a valuable medical tool, and the same is true, I suspect, about Electrosleep, though it has not yet won general acceptance either in Britain or the States. Ian Oswald, in his British Medical Association pamphlet Sleeping and Not Sleeping, *writes:*

"Electrosleep machines have never been proved to do any good," and elsewhere he has commented tartly: *"Some people just love magic boxes!"* Clearly a lot of questions remain to be answered. But the successes reported by Luce and Segal in the following chapter cannot be lightly dismissed.

〰〰〰〰〰〰〰〰〰〰〰〰〰〰〰〰〰〰〰〰

On an informal sun porch in a Jerusalem psychiatric hospital, a slender man with a graying beard and haunted dark eyes took off his glasses and lay down on a bed in his street clothes. . . . A nurse adjusted over his forehead a simple band containing some electrodes and wires. She flicked a switch on a gadget that might have been a small ham-radio transmitter. The man's face relaxed and he closed his eyes. A mild current was being diffused into his brain. . . . This man had seen his entire family killed by the Nazis. He had neither relaxed nor slept well since. Now, for the first time in twenty years, he was beginning to restore the normal pattern of nightly sleep. He was one of forty insomniacs, many of whom were addicted to drugs, who were beginning to return to normal life as a result of an experiment in electrosleep.

The Soviet Union has more than three hundred special clinics using electrotherapy routinely for a vast and astounding gamut of ailments. Is it possible that a single therapy could benefit them all—the obsessed insomniac, the child with asthma, the woman with ulcers, the man with hypertension, the boy with eczema, sufferers from muscle spasms, pregnancy toxemia, anxiety, depression, gastritis, colitis, and a few dozen other ailments? Could the same device prolong sleep for an insomniac but compress into half time the usual sleep of an ambitious young computer programmer? It sounds implausible at first, and doctors have developed an understandable skepticism about universal remedies, especially when they require expensive instruments. The more universal the claim, the less plausible a treatment will seem.

Twenty years ago the Russians began developing methods of electrical brain stimulation for anesthesia and sleep and evolved an instrument that came to be known as the Electroson. In translation, this was "electrosleep." Although there are many variations on the instrument itself, its basic purpose is to direct very mild electrical stimulation at lower regions of the brain. The frequency, the intensity of the electrical pulses, and the exact placement of the electrodes, have varied and must be carefully adjusted to each individual. Unlike electroshock therapy, in which the magnitude of the current induces convulsions, coma, and confusion, this mild stimulation seems to leave most people with no aftereffects at all. According to report, it has become almost a routine therapy in the Soviet Union.

Within the United States, this instrument has not been evaluated. Indeed, until recently, it was dismissed as quackery. Because of its name, the "electrosleep" instrument was expected to induce sleep. Researchers who tried it during the early 1960s were disappointed because it failed to put people to sleep. One Brooklyn researcher tried the instrument on about a hundred people, of whom only about half went to sleep. Nonetheless, many of them got up after their treatments feeling refreshed, calm, and alert, and a number of patients noticed that their usual muscle spasms had been diminished. Perhaps if the instrument had been called an Electric Tranquilizer, these beneficial side effects might have attracted some attention. Today, it is reasonably clear that electrosleep is a misnomer. The benefits of the treatment do not depend upon producing sleep at the time of stimulation. Still, there was historical reason why American medical scientists expected the machine to produce sleep.

Scientists throughout the world have been putting animals into instant sleep for many years by direct electrical stimulations of their brains. Their purpose was to find out which regions of the brain controlled sleep. They found not one or two regions but many. In each spot, stimulation had a strikingly different effect. One California researcher, for example, turned on a small current as a cat, with electrodes implanted in a spot inside his brain, was about to throttle a mouse. The cat dropped the mouse and sleepily retreated into a corner, where it curled up for a nap. Stimulation to a different region caused another cat, in the midst of hungrily eating his dinner, to drop asleep right into his food dish; yet, stimulation to another brain region caused only a light drowsing. There was no doubt in anyone's mind that electrical stimulation could cause sleep.

One of the puzzles with electrosleep, however, has been the variety of reactions seen in the normal people who have tried it. Some people sleep during the treatment; others do not. Some sleep more at night after treatment; others sleep less. Electrosleep has even caused severe nightmares in one test subject.

Once again, this variety of reactions would not seem surprising if we took account of brain research. The needlelike electrode that causes sleep when it discharges electric current at its tip need be moved only a microscopic distance —and now the current does not cause an animal to doze, but to snarl in evident rage. The duration or the frequency of electrical pulses, without moving the electrode, will cause different reactions, too; fast pulses may lead to arousal, while slow ones cause torpor. All this variation can occur from stimulating only one very tiny spot in the brain. We should not be surprised, then, that there is variation with electrosleep current, for this comes from outside the skull. The impulses cannot be aimed precisely at a few brain cells, and therefore nobody can be certain exactly where the current goes.

The explanation of effects from electrosleep may come from further research on animals and from recordings that are made on human patients before brain surgery. These researches are now going on in the Soviet Union, in France, Germany, and Israel. When a person takes an electrosleep treatment, is he enjoying direct electrical stimulation of his brain? Or does the current cause a change in brain circulation, or in chemistry?

Could the results have been the effect of suggestion? In one study of 2,500 patients, only 1,000 received any current during their treatment. They were then compared with the 1,500 who received no current at all. According to report, there was observable improvement among the people who received electrical stimulation, but no sign of change among the others. Evidently it was not mere suggestion that was at work.

Could there be some common link between all the ailments treated by "electrosleep"—from insomnia to asthma and hypertension? None are organic diseases; neither are they caused by infection or by a defect in a part of the body. In some sense, one might say that they all originate in the nervous system, whose governor is the brain. Within the brain, cells that invoke sleep lie near stations that regulate every aspect of our being—our moods, our blood circulation and pressure, digestive juices, hormones, pain perception, and, indeed, behavior. If ailments said to improve after electrosleep therapy are ailments of the nervous system, it seems plausible that the symptoms suffered could all be linked to a changing level of brain excitation or perhaps changes in the levels of crucial chemicals within certain brain regions.

One of the most careful and encouraging studies of electrosleep to date was inspired and designed by Florella Magora, an anesthesiologist at Hadassah Hospital in Jerusalem. She and her associates have demonstrated lasting improvements in insomniac patients, in asthmatic children, and many other patients. Nonetheless, Dr. Magora frequently comments, "We are not certain what it is we are doing yet."

Using an instrument that was designed at the hospital, they began trying the stimulation on fifteen healthy volunteers and three patients with Parkinsonian tremors or muscle spasms. The tremors of Parkinson's disease are known to vanish during sleep, and indeed, the two patients with this long and trying illness showed a complete disappearance of all symptoms after the current had been turned on. This was an encouraging sign, that the technique was producing natural sleep. Occasionally they would leave the current off. Now the person remained awake. When they turned the current on, he fell asleep. In many of their trials they seemed to be producing just what they hoped—electrically induced sleep.

However, there were seven healthy volunteers who didn't sleep. Some of them acted drowsy. They lay passively with their eyes closed, apparently drifting off, or at least losing grip on their conversational exchanges with the doctors. They said they had felt very pleasant and quite detached. Others who have experienced electrosleep, including one of the authors, make similar comments. One seems suspended. There are images flitting across the mind, and even dream fragments, experienced while listening to conversations and movements in the room. One has the impression that it would be possible to snap to attention instantly, while at the same time pervaded by a kind of laziness in which even speech seems an unnecessary effort. There is little impulse to talk or answer questions. At the end of treatment one is relaxed and fresh as after sleep, even if one did not sleep.

The Hadassah research team puzzled unhappily about their wakeful volunteers. Perhaps the electrodes had been wrongly placed and current had failed to penetrate a crucial brain region, or perhaps the current should have been increased for these people.

They now began to look at psychiatric patients who had suffered from insomnia for several years and for whom conventional remedies had not worked, and they also studied a group of asthmatic children who were not responding to conventional treatment. Once again, the medical team witnessed striking improvements even when people did not fall asleep during treatment.

If they worried that the effect was due to suggestion, the doctors were encouraged by the reaction of the children. They slept easily and could be calmed in the midst of a tantrum. One little girl, already wired, saw Dr. Magora approach with a syringe of water for wetting the electrodes and immediately began screaming in terror. She jumped up and howled. Dr. Magora turned on the current, and the child stopped shrieking, calmed down, and went to sleep. Asthmatic children who had been wheezing badly stopped during and after the treatment. Three of them were free of symptoms after four months. One child relapsed two months later, while the other two seemed to have improved. When the doctors tested for the effects of suggestion by leaving the current off, they found that these "dead" sessions produced no improvement in the children.

If the benefits of electrosleep seemed to have been transient among many asthmatic children, there were some strikingly lasting effects among the insomniacs. Twenty volunteers were especially selected for their severe and long-lasting insomnia. Four of them were young, between twenty-eight and thirty-eight, and the others were middle-aged and older. Several were selected because of their anxiety, their obsessiveness, depression, and addiction to barbiturates or morphine. All of them were taking sleeping pills; some were used to as much as a gram of barbiturate each night and would be tortured by withdrawal symptoms when the drug was removed. However, drugs were withheld before the beginning of the treatments.

Ten or more sessions were given, usually in the evening, for an hour or two. A number of people did not fall asleep initially when the current was turned on, but only five people seemed to be unaffected by the treatment. Slowly the normal pattern of normal sleep seemed to be returning. Some of the patients had been awakening from sleep without feeling refreshed, no matter how long they had slept. Others had become agitated and afraid at the fall of darkness, as if trying to do battle with an internal enemy that was escaping control. Others, typically, had awakened fretful and miserable at four or five in the morning. As they began to resume the habit of nightly sleep, their anxiety, depression, and withdrawal symptoms vanished, their gastritis and colitis diminished, and the whole group was able to leave the hospital. A follow-up, continued for twelve months, showed no relapses. The initial group of twenty patients was too small for general conclusions, yet again the improvement was too dramatic to be ignored.

At the end of 1967, forty patients had been taking treatment. Although their insomnia sprang from very different psychological sources and assumed various forms, the treatment seemed to work. It worked for an obsessed man for whom the onset of darkness brought back memories of his family's slaughter. It worked for engineers whose professional pressures caused them to drive themselves mercilessly. It worked for a woman in deep depression during pregnancy.

Several people, who began as subjects in an experiment, have requested a return visit for more. Word of the experiments with electrosleep began to spread after the publication of a popular article: two El Al pilots wanted to try the treatments themselves. They found that after a twelve-hour flight to the United States, they would lie in bed exhausted, but unable to sleep, and the incessant crossing of time zones was beginning to become a torture.

One of the many conjectures about the effectiveness of electrosleep suggests that the current, given at a fixed time of day, may be resynchronizing an individual's internal rhythms, like winding a clock. In experiments at the Institute of Living in Hartford, Connecticut, Charles Stroebel is studying the effects of electrosleep currents upon abnormal behavior and temperature rhythms in monkeys. There is some small evidence that very depressed people show disturbances in the daily rhythm of certain hormones. Other scientists have speculated that the current may be discharging some built-up excitement in the brain. It is pure speculation, yet research by William Dement and others suggests that this may be plausible. For instance, patients in hospitals have shown a decline in REM sleep after electroshock therapy. Would electrosleep therapy also reduce the amount of REM dreaming that a person required? Is it discharging the same chemical excitement?

Because we still do not understand the mechanisms that cause natural sleep, or the action of electrosleep, it seems unlikely that we could abolish sleep with current. Nonetheless, one young computer programmer has found that he was able to manage on an average of four and one half hours of sleep a night after taking daily treatments for thirty days. He had volunteered as an experimental subject at the Institute of Living. He reported to the laboratory regularly, like clockwork, each day. He soon commented that he enjoyed the treatment. It made him feel vital and healthy. Stroebel wondered if this might be the effect of exuberance, and occasionally throughout the next weeks would leave the current off. On these occasions the man would complain that something wasn't working. He would come in disgruntled the next day, complaining of fatigue. As the weeks went on, the man's nightly sleep was half of what he ordinarily required. He had taken on a second job, and was moonlighting with ease. By the end of seven weeks, he was thinking of electrosleep treatments as a way of life. At the end of nine weeks, although he showed no ill effects, it was decided that he should terminate treatments to see if the effect persisted. Rather quickly over a period of only a week he began to require his former quota of eight to nine hours of sleep in order to function efficiently.

Was the treatment making his sleep more efficient and restorative? Or was the current affecting a different region in this man's brain than the areas stimulated for prolonging sleep? It may take several years before there are answers. Now that the research has begun, we should begin to learn why electrosleep works and how to use the technique as an alternative to drugs. Perhaps the sleep clinic of the future may make little use of pills and syringes. It may instead be an electric dormitory to which insomniacs and other kinds of patients come for treatment at different hours of day or night. In the Soviet Union this idea is an actuality, and it is also being put to use in Austria and Israel. Strange as it may sound, the electric dormitory is not science fiction.

A Sleep Questionnaire

This questionnaire was devised by psychiatrists to assist them in diagnosing the kind of insomnia a patient might have. But it can also be used by an insomniac to help him evaluate his own sleep needs. There are no prizes for the right answers—and there aren't any wrong ones. But focusing on questions we don't normally ask ourselves about our habits of sleep can be a valuable exercise: the more we understand, the more likely we are to be reconciled to our personal insomniac difficulties.

～～～～～～～～～～～～～～～～～～～～～～～～

How many hours' sleep do you usually get? ☐ Has that changed? ☐ Since when?_____

How do you usually sleep?_____ Have you noticed any recent changes
in your sleep? ☐ If so, what kind?_____ Since when? _____

Do you always go to bed around the same time? ☐

What time do you go to bed nowadays? ☐ Is this earlier than it used to be?
☐ Later? ☐ If so, since when has this been happening? _____

Do you do (eat, drink, exercise) anything special before going to bed? _____

How long does it take you to fall asleep once you get to bed?_____ Has
it always taken that long? ☐ If not, since when has this been happening?

_____

Do you sleep best in a dark, quiet room ☐ or with radio on ☐ and lights
☐ ?

Do you wake up during the night? ☐ If so, how many times do you wake up?
☐ What time(s) do you wake up—more in the beginning of the night ☐
or more toward morning ☐ ? How long do you stay up?_____ How
long does it take you to fall asleep again? _____

Were you a good sleeper as a child? ☐ Where (with whom) did you sleep as
a child? _____

When did you last sleep through the whole night? _____

How is your memory? _____

What time do you wake up in the morning?_____ Do you get out of bed
right away? ☐ How do you feel when you awaken?_____ Do you
know right away that you are no longer asleep? ☐ Is this pattern the way
it has always been? ☐ If not, how did it used to be and when did this
change? _____

Do you take naps during the day? ☐ How long?_____ How often?__

_____ Is this your usual pattern? ☐ If not, when did this change?_____
_____ Do you exercise—at all ☐ a lot ☐ a little ☐ ?

Do you dream? ☐ If so, how often?_____ Is this the same as it has always been? ☐ If not, when did this change? _____

Do you dream as you are falling asleep? ☐

What do you dream about?_____ Do you dream about things in the present ☐ or the past ☐ ? Do you have nightmares? ☐ How often?_____
_____ Do you dream in color? ☐ Do you ever confuse your dreams with your waking state? ☐ Is all of this your usual pattern? ☐ If not, when did it change? _____

Do you take anything to help you sleep? ☐ If so, what?_____ Since when?_____ Do you take any alcohol after 7 P.M.? ☐ Have you always? ☐ If not, since when have you done so?_____ Have you needed more alcohol or medication to help you sleep recently? ☐ Since when?_____ How do drugs or alcohol affect your performance the next day?_____ What other medication or drugs have you been taking? _____

What time did you go to bed last night?_____ Did you take any medicine to help you sleep? ☐ How long did it take you to fall asleep?_____
_____ Did you wake up during the night? ☐ At what time(s)?_____
How long did it take you to fall asleep again?_____ What time did you wake up this morning?_____ Did you get up right away? ☐ If not, what time did you get up?_____ Did you dream last night? ☐
What about?_____ Was it pleasant? ☐ Did you take a nap today? ☐ If so, at what time(s)?_____ For how long?_____

Do you use an alarm clock? ☐ Do you wake up of your own accord? ☐

How do you react to alcohol—can you drink a lot without feeling it? ☐ Do you feel "high" on a drink or two? ☐

When you are feeling blue, do you find you like to go to sleep ☐ cannot sleep? ☐

What do you do when you are unable to sleep at night? _____

How seriously is your ability to cope with your work the following day affected by one or more bad nights? _____

Altered sleep patterns have been seen in hypothyroid, late pregnancy, retardation, depression, mental upset and psychosis, chronic brain syndrome, epilepsy, drug addiction, under steroid administration. Do you fit into any of these categories? _____

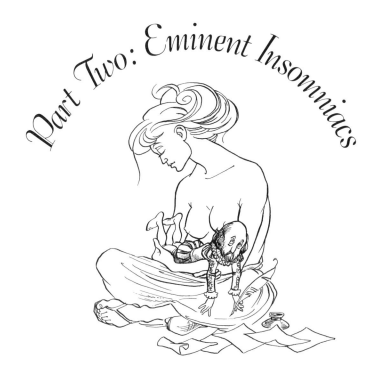

Part Two: Eminent Insomniacs

Shakespeare on Sleep

Although there are many references in classical literature to the virtues of sleep, there is hardly any writing of note—with one striking exception—about the opposite state of sleeplessness. We owe to Horace the famous phrase "I cannot sleep a wink," which we now know to be almost certainly either an exaggeration or a delusion.

The word "insomnia" itself only appears in the language in the middle of the eighteenth century, and it is not until fairly recently that the complaint appears to have become widespread. Might it be that insomnia is just one of the fashionable diseases of modern times? (However, if so, it is a fashion that shows no sign of losing its grip on its many millions of victims.) Whatever the reason, the topic is certainly a ubiquitous feature of contemporary diaries, journals, letters and essays.

The one striking exception is of course Shakespeare. The writings of Shakespeare abound with references to the subject of this book, and though he was a great borrower, none of his lines on sleep and insomnia can be traced to an earlier source.

Probably the most famous of all quotations about sleep is that from Macbeth:

> —the innocent sleep,
> Sleep that knits up the ravell'd sleave of care,
> The death of each day's life, sore labour's bath,
> Balm of hurt minds, great nature's second course,
> Chief nourisher in life's feast.

Dr. Hartmann has detected in this speech a prophetic insight on Shakespeare's part into REM and orthodox sleep. "Chief nourisher in life's feast" he identifies as a description of the restorative properties of delta sleep and as a preparation for the benefits of REM—"that knits up the ravell'd sleave of care."

Was Shakespeare an insomniac? His fascination with the subject, would incline one to think so until one remembers that he showed equal penetration on the subject (to name but three) of paranoia, senility or the Oedipus complex. If anyone is interested in pursuing the topic, I refer them to a little book entitled Shakespeare's Insomnia, *by Franklin H. Head, published in Boston in 1900. I don't think Dr. Head quite proves his case. Nevertheless, I make no apology for including Shakespeare in this section and for offering two of his most resonant passages on the subject, familiar though they may be to many readers.*

〜〜〜〜〜〜〜〜〜〜〜〜〜〜〜〜〜〜〜〜〜〜〜

> How many thousand of my poorest subjects
> Are at this hour asleep! O sleep, O gentle sleep,
> Nature's soft nurse, how have I frighted thee,
> That thou no more wilt weigh my eyelids down,

And steep my senses in forgetfulness?
Why rather, sleep, liest thou in smoky cribs,
Upon uneasy pallets stretching thee,
And hush'd with buzzing night-flies to thy slumber,
Than in the perfumed chambers of the great,
Under the canopies of costly state,
And lull'd with sound of sweetest melody?
O thou dull god, why liest thou with the vile
In loathsome beds, and leavest the kingly couch
A watch-case or a common 'larum-bell?
Wilt thou upon the high and giddy mast
Seal up the ship-boy's eyes, and rock his brains
In cradle of the rude imperious surge,
And in the visitation of the winds,
Who take the ruffian billows by the top,
Curling their monstrous heads, and hanging them
With deafening clamour in the slippery clouds,
That, with the hurly, death itself awakes?
Canst thou, O partial sleep, give thy repose
To the wet sea-boy in an hour so rude;
And in the calmest and most stillest night,
With all appliances and means to boot,
Deny it to a king? Then, happy low, lie down!
Uneasy lies the head that wears a crown.

                    II Henry IV, iii, 1

'Tis not the balm, the sceptre, and the ball,
The sword, the mace, the crown imperial,
The intertissued robe of gold and pearl,
The farced title running 'fore the king,
The throne he sits on, nor the tide of pomp
That beats upon the high shore of this world—
No, not all these, thrice gorgeous ceremony,
Not all these, laid in bed majestical,
Can sleep so soundly as the wretched slave,

Who, with a body fill'd and vacant mind
Gets him to rest, cramm'd with distressful bread;
Never sees horrid night, the child of hell;
But, like a lackey, from the rise to set
Sweats in the eye of Phoebus, and all night
Sleeps in Elysium . . .

Henry V, iv, 1

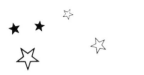

Overture

BY MARCEL PROUST

"Overture" is the name given by Proust to the opening pages of Swann's Way, itself the first volume of Remembrance of Things Past. *Like an operatic opener, this section rehearses what is to be a dominant theme of his work—the faculty of memory. I feel that recalling and exploring one's past, and perhaps especially one's memory of childhood, is more rewarding than most ways of spending insomniac hours. And if some readers find that Proust acts on them as a soporific —well,* tant mieux . . .

~~~~~~~~~~~~~~~~~~~~~~~~~~~~~~~~~~~~~

For a long time I used to go to bed early. Sometimes, when I had put out my candle, my eyes would close so quickly that I had not even time to say "I'm going to sleep." And half an hour later the thought that it was time to go to sleep would awaken me; I would try to put away the book which, I imagined, was still in my hands, and to blow out the light; I had been thinking all the time, while I was asleep, of what I had just been reading, but my thoughts had run into a channel of their own, until I myself seemed actually to have become the subject of my book: a church, a quartet, the rivalry between François I and Charles V. This impression would persist for some moments after I was awake; it did not disturb my mind, but it lay like scales upon my eyes and prevented them from registering the fact that the candle was no longer burning. Then it would begin to seem unintelligible, as the thoughts of a former existence must be to a reincarnate spirit; the subject of my book would separate itself from me, leaving me free to choose whether I would form part of it or no; and at the same time my sight would return and I would be astonished to find myself in a state of darkness, pleasant and restful enough for the eyes, and even more, perhaps, for my mind, to which it appeared incomprehensible, without a cause, a matter dark indeed.

I would ask myself what o'clock it could be; I could hear the whistling of trains, which, now nearer and now farther off, punctuating the distance like the note of a bird in a forest, shewed me in perspective the deserted countryside through which a traveller would be hurrying towards the nearest station: the path that he followed being fixed for ever in his memory by the general excitement due to being in a strange place, to doing unusual things, to the last words of conversation, to farewells exchanged beneath an unfamiliar lamp which echoed still in his ears amid the silence of the night; and to the delightful prospect of being once again at home.

I would lay my cheeks gently against the comfortable cheeks of my pillow, as plump and blooming as the cheeks of babyhood. Or I would strike a match to look at my watch. Nearly midnight. The hour when an invalid, who has been obliged to start on a journey and to sleep in a strange hotel, awakens in a moment of illness and sees with glad relief a streak of daylight shewing under his bedroom door. Oh, joy of joys! It is morning. The servants will be about in a minute: he can ring, and some one will come to look after him. The thought of being made comfortable gives him strength to endure his pain. He is certain he heard footsteps: they come nearer, and then die away. The ray of light beneath his door is extinguished. It is midnight; someone has turned out the gas; the last servant has gone to bed, and he must lie all night in agony with no one to bring him any help.

I would fall asleep, and often I would be awake again for short snatches only, just long enough to hear the regular creaking of the wainscot, or to open my eyes to settle the shifting kaleidoscope of the darkness, to savour, in an instantaneous flash of perception, the sleep which lay heavy upon the furniture, the room, the whole surroundings of which I formed but an insignificant part and whose unconsciousness I should very soon return to share. Or, perhaps, while I was asleep I had returned without the least effort to an earlier stage in my life, now for ever outgrown; and had come under the thrall of one of my childish terrors, such as that old terror of my great-uncle's pulling my curls, which was effectually dispelled on the day— the dawn of a new era to me—on which they were finally cropped from my head. I had forgotten that event during my sleep; I remembered it again immediately I had succeeded in making myself wake up to escape my great-uncle's fingers; still, as a measure of precaution, I would bury the whole of my head in the pillow before returning to the world of dreams.

Sometimes, too, just as Eve was created from a rib of Adam, so a woman would come into existence while I was sleeping, conceived from some strain in the position of my limbs. Formed by the appetite that I was on the point of gratifying, she it was, I imagined, who offered me that gratification. My body, conscious that its own warmth was permeating hers, would strive to become one with her, and I would awake. The rest of humanity seemed very remote in comparison with this woman whose company I had left but a moment ago: my cheek was still warm with her kiss, my body bent beneath the weight of hers. If, as would sometimes happen, she had the appearance of some woman whom I had known in waking hours, I would abandon myself altogether to the sole quest of her, like people who set out on a journey to see with their own eyes some city that they have always longed to visit, and imagine that they can taste in reality what has charmed their fancy. And then, gradually, the memory of her would dissolve and vanish, until I had forgotten the maiden of my dream.

When a man is asleep, he has in a circle round him the chain of the hours, the sequence of the years, the order of the heavenly host. Instinctively, when he awakes, he looks to these, and in an instant reads off his own position on the earth's surface and the amount of time that has elapsed during his slumbers; but this ordered procession is apt to grow confused, and to break its ranks. Suppose that, towards morning, after a night of insomnia, sleep descends upon him while he is reading, in quite a different position from that in which he normally goes to sleep, he has only to lift his arm to arrest the sun and turn it back in its course, and, at the moment of waking, he will have no idea of the time, but will conclude that he has just gone to bed. Or suppose that he gets drowsy in some even more abnormal position; sitting in an armchair, say, after dinner: then the world will fall topsy-turvy from its orbit, the magic chair will carry him at full speed through time and space, and when he opens his eyes again he will imagine that he went to sleep months earlier and in some far distant country. But for me it was enough if, in my own bed, my sleep was so heavy as completely to relax my consciousness; for then I lost all sense of the place in which I had gone to sleep, and when I awoke at midnight, not knowing where I was, I could not be sure at first who I was; I had only the most rudimentary sense of existence, such as may lurk and flicker in the depths of an animal's consciousness; I was more destitute of human qualities than the cave dweller; but then the memory, not yet of the place in which I was, but of various other places where I had lived, and might now very possibly be, would come like a rope let down from heaven to draw me up out of the abyss of not-being, from which I could never have escaped by myself: in a flash I would traverse and surmount centuries of civilisation, and out of a half-visualised succession of oil-lamps, followed by shirts with turned-down collars, would put together by degrees the component parts of my ego.

Rejected by Sleep

BY FRANZ KAFKA

If insomnia is a paradigm malady of our times, Kafka, with his chronic neuras-
thenia and his painful sense of alienation, may stand as a paradigm insomniac.
His diaries return again and again to the subject. Here, writing in his Diary for
1911, he describes two sleepless nights which, though tormenting, serve to
confirm his confidence in his creative genius.

October 2. Sleepless night. The third in a row. I fall asleep soundly, but after
an hour I wake up, as though I had laid my head in the wrong hole. I am
completely awake, have the feeling that I have not slept at all or only under
a thin skin, have before me anew the labour of falling asleep and feel myself

rejected by sleep . . . Toward morning I sigh into the pillow, because for this night all hope is gone. I think of those nights at the end of which I was raised out of deep sleep and awoke as though I had been folded in a nut.

I believe this sleeplessness comes only because I write. For no matter how little and how badly I write, I am still made sensitive by these minor shocks, feel, especially toward evening and even more in the morning, the approaching, the imminent possibility of great moments which would tear me open, which could make me capable of anything, and in the general uproar that is within me and which I have no time to command, find no rest. In the end this uproar is only a suppressed, restrained harmony, which, left free, would fill me completely, which could even widen me and yet still fill me. But now such a moment arouses only feeble hopes and does me harm, for my being does not have sufficient strength or the capacity to hold the present mixture; during the day the visible world helps me, during the night it cuts me to pieces unhindered.

October 3. The same sort of night, but fell asleep with even more difficulty. While falling asleep a vertically moving pain in my head over the bridge of the nose, as though from a wrinkle too sharply pressed into my forehead. To make myself as heavy as possible, which I consider good for falling asleep, I had crossed my arms and laid my hands on my shoulders, so that I lay there like a soldier with his pack. Again it was the power of my dreams, shining forth into wakefulness even before I fall asleep, which did not let me sleep. In the evening and the morning my consciousness of the creative abilities in me is more than I can encompass. I feel shaken to the core of my being and can get out of myself whatever I desire.

On Board the SS Caliban

BY EVELYN WAUGH

Self-pity is an abiding temptation for insomniacs, and naturally a dominant feature of much insomniac writing. It is at its reeking worst, for instance, in the lugubrious poem "Insomnia" by the nineteenth-century poet James Thomson (sometimes called "the laureate of pessimism"):

> But I with infinite weariness outworn,
> > Haggard with endless nights unblessed by sleep,
> Ravaged by thoughts unutterably forlorn,
> > Plunged in despairs unfathomably deep,
> Went cold and pale and trembling with affright
> Into the desert vastitude of Night,
> > Arid and wild and black;
> Foreboding no oasis of sweet slumber,
> Counting beforehand all the countless number
> Of sands that are its minutes on my desolate track.

But not all insomniac writers burden readers with their grievances. One doesn't need the evidence of Evelyn Waugh's posthumous diaries to realize that he suffered cruelly from insomnia, aggravated by an assortment of powerful sleeping pills and alcohol. (Marilyn Monroe and Judy Garland are two other notable victims of the same poisonous combination.) His astonishingly self-revealing novel The Ordeal of Gilbert Pinfold, *from which these extracts are taken, not only stands as a fearful warning of the hallucinations that can follow when an insomniac mixes drinks and drugs, but also as a memorial to Waugh's stoic acceptance of his disability.*

〰〰〰〰〰〰〰〰〰〰〰〰〰〰〰〰〰〰〰〰〰

Mr. Pinfold slept badly. It was a trouble of long standing. For twenty-five years he had used various sedatives, for the last ten years a single specific, chloral and bromide which, unknown to Dr. Drake, he bought on an old prescription in London. There were periods of literary composition when he would find the sentences he had written during the day running in his head, the words shifting and changing colour kaleidoscopically, so that he would again and again climb out of bed, pad down to the library, make a minute correction, return to his room, lie in the dark dazzled by the pattern of vocables until obliged once more to descend to the manuscript. But those days and nights of obsession, of what might without vainglory be called 'creative' work, were a small part of his year. On most nights he was neither fretful nor apprehensive. He was merely bored. After even the idlest day he demanded six or seven hours of insensibility. With them behind him, with them to look forward to, he could face another idle day with something approaching jauntiness; and these his doses unfailingly provided.

The composition of his sleeping-draught, as originally prescribed, was largely of water. He suggested to his chemist that it would save trouble to have the essential ingredients in full strength and to dilute them himself. Their taste was bitter and after various experiments he found they were most palatable in creme de menthe. He was not scrupulous in measuring the dose. He splashed into the glass as much as his mood suggested and if he took too little and woke in the small hours he would get out of bed and make unsteadily for the bottles and a second swig. Thus he passed many hours in welcome unconsciousness; but all was not well with him. Whether from too much strong medicine or from some other cause, he felt decidedly seedy by the middle of November. He found himself disagreeably flushed, particularly after drinking his normal, not illiberal, quantity of wine and brandy. Crimson blotches appeared on the back of his hands.

He called in Dr. Drake, who said: "That sounds like an allergy."

"Allergic to what?"

"Ah, that's hard to say. Almost anything can cause an allergy nowadays. It might be something you're wearing or some plant growing near. The only cure really is a change."

"I might go abroad after Christmas."

"Yes, that's the best thing you could do. Anyway, don't worry. No one ever died of an allergy. It's allied to hayfever," he added learnedly, "and asthma."

Another thing which troubled him and which he soon began to attribute to his medicine was the behaviour of his memory. It began to play him tricks. He did not grow forgetful. He remembered everything in clear detail but he remembered it wrong. He would state a fact, dogmatically, sometimes in print —a date, a name, a quotation—find himself challenged, turn to his books for verification and find most disconcertingly that he was at fault.

After one or two alarming incidents, Pinfold is advised for his health's sake to take a sea voyage. Here is his first night out on the SS Caliban:

He noticed his grey pills, took one, lay down, opened his book, and then to the sound of dance tunes fell asleep once more.

Perhaps he dreamed. He forgot on the instant whatever had happened in the hours between. It was dark. He was awake and there was a very curious scene being played near him; under his feet, it seemed. He heard distinctly a clergyman conducting a religious meeting. Mr. Pinfold had no first-hand acquaintance with evangelical practice. His home and his schools had professed a broad-to-high anglicanism. His ideas of nonconformity derived from literature, from Mr. Chadband and Philip Henry Gosse, from charades and from back numbers of *Punch.* The sermon, which was just rising to its peroration, was plainly an expression of that kind of faith, scriptural in diction, emotional in appeal. It was addressed presumably to members of the crew. Male voices sang a hymn which Mr. Pinfold remembered from his nursery where his nanny, like almost all nannies, had been Calvinist: *"Pull for the shore, sailor. Pull for the shore."*

"I want to see Billy alone after you dismiss," said the clergyman. There followed an extempore, rather perfunctory prayer, then a great shuffling of feet and pushing about of chairs; then a hush; then the clergyman, very earnestly: "Well, Billy, what have you got to say to me?" and the unmistakable sound of sobbing.

Mr. Pinfold began to feel uneasy. This was something that was not meant to be overheard.

"Billy, you must tell me yourself. I am not accusing you of anything. I am not putting words into your mouth."

Silence except for sobbing.

"Billy, you know what we talked about last time. Have you done it again? Have you been impure, Billy?"

"Yes, sir. I can't help it, sir."

"God never tempts us beyond our strength, Billy. I've told you that, haven't I? Do you suppose I do not feel these temptations, too, Billy? Very strongly at times. But I resist, don't I? You know I resist, don't I, Billy?"

Mr. Pinfold was horror-struck. He was being drawn into participation in a scene of gruesome indecency. His sticks lay by the bunk. He took the black-thorn and beat strongly on the floor.

"Did you hear anything then, Billy? A knocking. That is God knocking at the door of your soul. He can't come and help you unless you are pure, like me."

This was more than Mr. Pinfold could bear. He took painfully to his feet, put on his coat, brushed his hair. The voices below him continued:

"I can't help it, sir. I want to be good. I try. I can't."

"You've got pictures of girls stuck up by your bunk, haven't you?"

"Yes, sir."

"How can you say you want to be good when you keep temptation deliberately before your eyes. I shall come and destroy those pictures."

"No, please, sir. I want them."

Mr. Pinfold hobbled out of his cabin and up to the main deck. The sea was calmer now. More passengers were about in the lounge and the bar. It was half past six. A group were throwing dice for drinks. Mr. Pinfold sat alone and ordered a cocktail. When the steward brought it, he asked: "Does this ship carry a regular chaplain?"

"Oh no, sir. The Captain reads the prayers on Sundays."

"There's a clergyman, then, among the passengers?"

"I haven't seen one, sir. Here's the list."

Mr. Pinfold studied the passenger list. No name bore any prefix indicating Holy Orders. A strange ship, though Mr. Pinfold, in which laymen were allowed to evangelize a presumably heathen crew; religious mania perhaps on the part of one of the officers.

After dinner the following night, Pinfold retires early to his cabin.

It was not yet nine o'clock. Mr. Pinfold undressed. He hung up his clothes, washed, and took his pill. There were three tablespoonfuls left in his bottle of sleeping-draught. He decided to try and spend the night without it, to delay anyway until after midnight. The sea was much calmer now; he could lie in bed without rolling. He lay at ease and began to read one of the novels he had brought on board.

Then, before he had turned a page, the band struck up. This was no wireless performance. It was a living group just under his feet, rehearsing. They were in the same place, as inexplicably audible, as the afternoon bible-class; young happy people, the party doubtless from the purser's table. Their instruments were drums and rattles and some sort of pipe. The drums and rattles did most of the work. Mr. Pinfold knew nothing of music. It seemed to him that the rhythms they played derived from some very primitive tribe and were of anthropological rather than artistic interest. This guess was confirmed.

"Let's try the Pocoputa Indian one," said the young man who acted, without any great air of authority, as leader.

"Oh not *that.* It's so *beastly,*" said a girl.

"I know," said the leader. "It's the three-eight rhythm. The Gestapo discovered it independently, you know. They used to play it in the cells. It drove the prisoners mad."

"Yes," said another girl. "Thirty-six hours did for anyone. Twelve was enough for most. They could stand any torture but that."

"It drove them absolutely mad." "Raving mad." "Stark, staring mad." "It was the worst torture of all." "The Russians use it now." The voices, some male, some female, all young and eager, came tumbling like puppies. "The Hungarians do it best." "Good old three-eight." "Good old Pocoputa Indians." "They were mad."

"I suppose no one can hear us?" said a sweet girlish voice.

"Don't be so wet, Mimi. Everyone's up on the main deck."

"All right then," said the band leader. "The three-eight rhythm."

And off they went.

The sound throbbed and thrilled in the cabin which had suddenly become a prison cell. Mr. Pinfold was not one who thought and talked easily to a musical accompaniment. Even in early youth he had sought the night-clubs where there was a bar out of hearing of the band. Friends he had, Roger Stillingfleet among them, to whom jazz was a necessary drug—whether stimulant or narcotic Mr. Pinfold did not know. He preferred silence. The three-eight rhythm was indeed torture to him. He could not read. It was not a quarter of an hour since he had entered the cabin. Unendurable hours lay ahead. He emptied the bottle of sleeping-draught and, to the strains of the jolly young people from the purser's table, fell into unconsciousness.

He awoke before dawn. The bright young people below him had dispersed. The three-eight rhythm was hushed. No shadow passed between the deck-light and the cabin-window. But overhead there was turmoil. The crew, or a considerable part of it, was engaged on an operation of dragging the deck with what from the sound of it might have been an enormous chain-harrow, and they were not happy in their work. They were protesting mutinously in their own tongue and the officer in command was roaring back at them in the tones of an old sea-dog: "Get on with it, you black bastards. Get on with it."

The lascars were not so easily quelled. They shouted back unintelligibly.

"I'll call out the Master-at-Arms," shouted the officer. An empty threat, surely? thought Mr. Pinfold. It was scarcely conceivable that the *Caliban* carried a Master-at-Arms. "By God, I'll shoot the first man of you that moves," said the officer.

The hubbub increased. Mr. Pinfold could almost see the drama overhead, the half-lighted deck, the dark frenzied faces, the solitary bully with the heavy old-fashioned ship's pistol. Then there was a crash, not a shot but a huge percussion of metal as though a hundred pokers and pairs of tongs had fallen into an enormous fender, followed by a wail of agony and a moment of complete silence.

"There," said the officer more in the tones of a nanny than a sea-dog. "Just see what you've gone and done now."

Whatever its nature this violent occurrence entirely subdued the passions of the crew. They were docile, ready to do anything to retrieve the disaster. The only sounds now were the officer's calmer orders and the whimpering of the injured man.

"Steady there. Easy does it. You, cut along to the sick-bay and get the surgeon. You, go up and report to the bridge . . ."

For a long time, two hours perhaps, Mr. Pinfold lay in his bunk, listening. He was able to hear quite distinctly not only what was said in his immediate vicinity, but elsewhere. He had the light on, now, in his cabin, and as he gazed at the complex of tubes and wires which ran across his ceiling, he realized that they must form some kind of general junction in the system of communication. Through some trick or fault or wartime survival everything spoken in the executive quarters of the ship was transmitted to him. When she was a naval vessel this cabin had no doubt been the office of some operational headquarters and when she was handed back to her owners and re-adapted for passenger service, the engineers had neglected to disconnect it. That alone could explain the voices which now kept him informed of every stage of the incident.

The wounded man seemed to have got himself entangled in some kind of web of metal. Various unsuccessful and agonizing attempts were made to extricate him. Finally the decision was taken to cut him out. The order once given was carried out with surprising speed but the contraption, whatever it was, was ruined in the process and was finally dragged across the deck and thrown overboard. The victim continuously sobbed and whimpered. He was taken to the sick-bay and put in charge of a kind but not, it appeared, very highly qualified nurse. "You must be brave," she said. "I will say the rosary for you. You must be brave," while the wireless telegraphist got into touch with a hospital ashore and was given instructions in first-aid. The ship's surgeon never appeared. Details of treatment were dictated from the shore and passed to the sick-bay. The last words Mr. Pinfold heard from the bridge were Captain Steerforth's "I'm not going to be bothered with a sick man on board. We'll have to signal a passing homebound ship and have him transferred."

Part of the treatment prescribed by the hospital was a sedative injection, and as this spread its relief over the unhappy lascar, Mr. Pinfold too grew drowsy until finally he fell asleep to the sound of the nurse murmuring the Angelic Salutation.

He was awakened by the coloured cabin steward bringing him tea.

"Very disagreeable business that last night," said Mr. Pinfold.

"Yes, sir."

"How is the poor fellow?"

"Eight o'clock, sir."

"Have they managed to get into touch with a ship to take him off?"

"Yes, sir. Breakfast eight-thirty, sir."

Mr. Pinfold drank his tea. He felt disinclined to get up. The intercommunication system was silent. He picked up his book and began to read. Then with a click the voices began again.

Captain Steerforth seemed to be addressing a deputation of the crew. "I want you to understand," he was saying, "that a great quantity of valuable metal was sacrificed last night for the welfare of a single seaman. That metal was pure *copper*. One of the most valuable metals in the world. Mind you I don't regret the sacrifice and I am sure the Company will approve my action. But I want you all to appreciate that only in a British ship would such a thing be done. In the ship of any other nationality it would have been the seaman not the metal that was cut up. You know that as well as I do. Don't forget it. And another thing, instead of taking the man with us to Port Said and the filth of a Wog hospital, I had him carefully trans-shipped and he is now on his way to England. He couldn't have been treated more handsomely if he'd been a director of the Company. I know the hospital he's going to; it's a sweet, pretty place. It's the place all seamen long to go to. He'll have the best attention there and live, if he does live, in the greatest comfort. That's the kind of ship this is. Nothing is too good for the men who serve in her."

The meeting seemed to disperse. There was a shuffling and muttering and presently a woman spoke. It was a voice which was soon to become familiar to Mr. Pinfold. To all men and women there is some sound—grating, perhaps, or rustling, or strident, deep or shrill, a note or inflection of speech—which causes peculiar pain; which literally "makes the hair stand on end" or metaphorically "sets the teeth on edge"; something which Dr. Drake would have called an "allergy." Such was this woman's voice. It clearly did not affect the Captain in this way but to Mr. Pinfold it was excruciating.

"Well," said this voice. "That should teach them not to grumble."

"Yes," said Captain Steerforth. "We've settled that little mutiny, I think. We shouldn't have any trouble now."

"Not till the next time," said the cynical woman. "What a contemptible exhibition that man made of himself—crying like a child. Thank God we've seen the last of him. I liked your touch about the sweet, pretty hospital."

"Yes. They little know the Hell-spot I've sent him to. Spoiling my copper, indeed. He'll soon wish he were in Port Said."

And the woman laughed odiously. "Soon wish he was dead," she said.

There was a click (someone seemed to be in control of the apparatus, Mr. Pinfold thought), and two passengers were speaking. They seemed to be elderly, military gentlemen.

"I think the passengers should be told," one said.

"Yes, we ought to call a meeting. It's the sort of thing that so often passes without proper recognition. We ought to pass a vote of thanks."

"A ton of copper, you say?"

"Pure copper, cut up and chucked overboard. All for the sake of a nigger. It makes one proud of the British service."

The voices ceased and Mr. Pinfold lay wondering about this meeting; was it his duty to attend and report what he knew of the true characters of the Captain and his female associate? The difficulty, of course, would be to prove his charges; to explain satisfactorily how he came to overhear the Captain's secret.

Soft music filled the cabin, an oratorio sung by a great but distant choir. "That *must* be a gramophone record," thought Mr. Pinfold. "Or the wireless. They can't be performing this on board." Then he slept for some time, until he was woken by a change of music. The bright young people were at it again with their Pocoputa Indian three-eight rhythm. Mr. Pinfold looked at his watch. Eleven-thirty. Time to get up.

Before leaving his cabin he considered his box of pills. He was not too well. Much was wrong with him, he felt, beside lameness. Dr. Drake did not know about the sleeping-draught. It might be that the pills, admittedly new and pretty strong, warred with the bromide and chloral; perhaps with gin and brandy too. Well, the sleeping-draught was finished. He would try the pills once or twice more. He swallowed one and crept up to the main deck . . .

Part Three: Pursuing Sleep

Eighty-Two Tried and Proven Ways of Wooing Sleep

This section might be called a reconnaissance into an almost completely un-known region—the folklore of insomnia. In order to cast my net as widely as possible, I wrote letters to newspapers and magazines, and appeared on radio and television, inviting people to write to me. The response was tremendous. Many people took enormous trouble to explain in detail how they had cured or eased their insomnia, and I felt embarrassed at replying briefly to so much generous help. The letters, which came from young and old, from men and women, and from very simple to highly sophisticated correspondents, were a further reminder, if one was needed, of how widespread a complaint insomnia is. What follows is a selection of the most plausible and the most diverting—with a few tips from a handful of celebrities.

I have omitted from this part of the book perhaps the most popular "remedies" of all: the innumerable varieties of mental exercise connected with letters and numbers. You will find a précis of them in the chapter called Brain Games. *It is arguable whether playing with words and numbers really is a method of wooing sleep rather than of keeping the mind cheerful and distracted during the night. On the whole, though an inveterate midnight wordsmith myself, I am inclined to the latter view.*

Not surprisingly, many of the same remedies reappear again and again. Just as there are said to be no more than a dozen (or perhaps no more than four) different plots for would-be novelists, so you might say that there are only about seven or eight basic techniques available for intending sleepers. But each theme has many variations.

Many of the letters I received ended with some message such as "I can't recommend my method too highly. It's infallible." Maybe for that individual, but alas, just as everyone needs to find out for himself how many hours of sleep his own organism requires, so each insomniac must develop his own sleep-wooing rituals. When it comes to sleep, it's every man for himself.

〰〰〰〰〰〰〰〰〰〰〰〰〰〰〰〰〰

PLEASANT NIGHTTIME DAYDREAMS

You are a baby in a pram and someone is gently rocking you to sleep.

* * *

You are floating very gently on a soft, white, fleecy cloud. Murmur to yourself:

> Now fades the glimmering landscape on the night,
> And all the air a solemn stillness holds.

Save where the beetle wheels his droning flight,
And drowsy tinklings lull the distant folds.

* * *

Imagine situations that employ each of the five senses in turn, e.g.:

hearing: waves breaking on the sea shore, or favorite music
sight: pastoral scenes
smell: the scent of flowers
taste: favorite food or drink
touch: the warmth of the sun on your cheek or a cool breeze
through your hair

* * *

Retrace your steps on some special long walk.

* * *

You are at the controls of a large jet. The aircraft, packed with excited passengers, stands ready for takeoff, waiting for the control tower's radio command. All four mighty engines are on minimum power. Then, suddenly, by a mere flick of your wrist on the throttles, effortless thrust projects the slender beast along the runway. As the plane accelerates faster and faster, the electronics of this engineering masterpiece hum in complete unison. The instruments indicate takeoff speed. You pull back the control column and curve skyward. At an incredible angle of climb, you soar to 50,000 feet, the earth disappearing rapidly from view. As the aircraft continues to gather more and more speed, you level off. The clouds, now far below, appear to be moving backward. By the time you have skimmed through the sound barrier and passed 1,000 m.p.h., you are lulled to sleep by the solitude and majesty of the stratosphere.

* * *

Imagine yourself a bee creeping into different blooms, watching the colors on the gorgeous petals, then the thick stamens and the crop of honey.

* * *

As a very young child my family spent an entire summer on a farm in New Jersey. I was fascinated by everything I saw and learned. The thing that made a lasting impression was the lovely fragrance of the apple blossoms in the orchard. I recall that wonderful fragrance and in no time at all I fall asleep.

* * *

Imagine you are in a log cabin in Canada. Outside is thick snow, and the wolves are howling. But inside a fire protects you from the cold, and a stout door from the wolves. You are safe, warm and comfortable on a few blankets on the floor, and you have the cozy red light of your flickering fire.

* * *

Play through a game of golf in detail, counting the strokes.

* * *

When I turn out the light, I drift into the following fantasy: first, I seem to be no longer my real age (I was a schoolboy when Queen Victoria was celebrating her diamond jubilee in 1897) but about thirty years old—active and unencumbered by an ageing body. I seem to be enclosed in an invisible aura or cocoon which protects me from any harm. I cannot be shot at or stabbed. I am impervious to heat or cold. I can go out in freezing weather clad only in summer clothes. I can keep cool in a steaming jungle. In this fantasy, I can go back centuries in time, talk to historical celebrities, etc. No guard can hold me back. Now the marvellous part of this system of mine is that I am no more embarked on one of these adventures or astral flights, than it all fades and I am fast asleep.

Every night I do something different and it always works. Last night, for instance, I stood (in my imagination, of course) in front of an old mansion on 14th Street which no longer exists. I lived there over fifty years ago and at that time the landlady told me it had once been an elegant mansion. I saw it first as it was in 1920. Then I took off ten years and then another ten till I was back in

1840. By that time everything modern had gone and I saw what a beautiful neighbourhood it had been in those days. And by that time I was fast asleep.

*   *   *

Imagine yourself one of the great orchestras and become in turn a first violin or a French horn or a piece of percussion.

*   *   *

Years ago I tried to visualise the site where I would want to build a house. I often found it was morning before my spot was found. Over the years I improvised on this theme. I have built and furnished my four-bedroomed house, complete with maid; I have had landscape gardeners plan my garden and greenhouse. This planning was probably spread over four or five years, but the hard imaginative work invariably brought sleep. As I grew older, my four-bedroomed house became smaller as my children married and left home, and grew again as the grandchildren arrived. The garden became less ornamental and more utilitarian as places had to be found for swings and sandpits. Now that we are older, we have moved to a bungalow with a smaller garden. So now I spend my sleepless nights visualizing a glass-covered verandah on two sides of the bungalow, half to be a furnished sun-lounge, half for potted plants and seed boxes. Even if nothing comes of these plans, I certainly derive pleasure from imagining them; and sooner or later I fall asleep, and carry on with the next instalment on another occasion.

*   *   *

I treat myself like an infant in a pram, cuddle over in my favourite position which I call my "snoozle-doozle" position and recite to myself everything I did that day in order *or* count the calories I ate that day *or* think of my earliest impressions *or* go over floor-plans of houses I have lived in or visited *or* assemble clothing outfits, deciding what shoes, scarfs, etc., go together.

*   *   *

You are left a fortune and you plan to spend it.

*   *   *

Try to remember what you were doing on the same date a month or a year ago.

*   *   *

Describe your home village, town or city in the clearest possible terms, as though to a complete stranger.

TECHNIQUES OF CONCENTRATION

Having taken a full inspiration . . . the patient must depict to himself that he sees the breath passing from his nostrils in a continuous stream, and the very instant that he brings his mind to conceive this apart from all other ideas, consciousness and memory depart. For the instant the mind is brought to the contemplation of a single sensation, that instant the sensorium abdicates the throne and the hypnotic faculty steeps it in oblivion . . . Even should it not succeed in inducing very sound sleep, he will at least fall into that state of pleasing delirium which is a precursor of repose and which is scarcely inferior to it.
—Dr. Edward E. Binns,
Anatomy of Sleep, 1845

*   *   *

Imagine a room covered wall to wall and floor to ceiling with black velvet.

*   *   *

Concentrate on the blackness behind your closed eyelids. Imagine a yellow speck in the top left-hand corner of the darkness. Enter into the blackness and begin traveling steadily toward the speck, as though in a cave working your way toward the outside up a steep tunnel. Slowly approach the yellow patch until you can see the sky.

*   *   *

Visualize a large white sheet hanging on a line. Approach closer and closer until you can see nothing but the sheet. Concentrate on the weave so that all other thoughts are blotted out.

* * *

Make your mind a complete blank and think gray, like an overexposed negative. Prevent the gray from taking the shape of anything. If it does, switch back to gray at once—all the time breathing deeply and steadily.

* * *

Pretend that you are looking out at a very large, still lake located between your eyes.

* * *

Keep repeating "sleep, sleep, s l e e p, s l e e p"—until you drop off.

* * *

Imagine a hand very slowly and carefully drawing the number 3 on a completely black blackboard.

* * *

Picture a large figure 21. Now look at the 2 and "say" 1. Then regard the 1 and "say" 2. Repeat, and by about the fifth attempt you will be asleep.

* * *

Focus the mind between the two eyes and repeat a mantra over and over again. The mantra I use is *"Om tat sat"*—meaning in Sanskrit "Om that is good" or "Om that is real" or "Om that exists"—a description of the Supreme Spirit of Hinduism.

* * *

We need an inner warden to halt the nonstop traffic—the irrepressible and often nagging thoughts that accompany insomnia. To impose such a quietus successfully, the mind must be able to conceive of Emptiness and to retreat into it at will. Count the ticks of a clock, or any repetitive sound, then deliberately STOP your counting while continuing to listen to the beats. Interrupt a train of thought by consciously switching attention onto some quite unrelated matter or event of no interest at all. Go Blank, if only for a short moment at a time, but progressively for longer moments. Adopt a mnemonic to focus attention: the shape of the capital letters *M* and *T*. They have no significance in themselves, and should be obstinately held in thought by the conscious rejection of any intruding ideas, words or images. Think of *M* clearly, then of *T;* then join them as *MT*. The effect will be felt, punwisely, as *EMPTY*, a powerful switch into mind-emptiness. *MT* should be visualized while *"Empty"* is repeated again and again, like a needle stuck in a groove of a record. Practice will establish an ever quicker path to thought cessation, which is Emptiness, the precondition of Sleep.

* * *

Lie flat on your back, drop lower jaw to most relaxed position and listen to your breathing.

* * *

Imagine that your body is made of hollow glass. With each breath you draw in a cloudy mixture and exhale it through your body down to your toes. You repeat until your whole body is full of cloudy stuff. The deeper you breathe in, the more space you can fill, but it takes a long time to fill your thighs and toes.

* * *

Pretend that you are alone in a canoe in very rough seas. Breathe regularly, and quite deeply, in the way normal sleepers do. Each time you inhale, paddle the canoe. Sometimes the waves are very high and choppy, and paddling is difficult. But with each breath there is that paddle stroke, and the storm must be ridden out. Occasionally I let my canoe turn into a rowboat, and row instead of paddle. Sometimes I alternate: paddle/breath, row/breath, paddle/breath, row/breath . . . and before . . . I . . . know . . . it . . . the alarm goes . . . off . . . and . . . it . . . is . . . morning.

* * *

The important thing is to stop words. Focus the attention on a blank screen. If this is held—or returned to each time words return—images, not necessarily clear at first, will appear. These pictures must not be induced or recollected or simply remembered. They must be allowed to appear on the darkness which takes place from the effort of giving up the repetition of words. This exercise will remove the ordinary mechanical attention from the inner conversations about personal worries or daily affairs.

* * *

Numb the brain by requiring it to perform a dull, boring task, like repeating the words "Pooh" and "Bah" in ever-increasing numbers. The "Poohs" must always be two more than the "Bahs," giving the following sequence:

1. Pooh
2. Pooh Pooh Bah
3. Pooh Pooh Pooh Bah
4. Pooh Pooh Pooh Pooh Bah Bah
   —and so on.

If a mistake is made, or the number of words required is forgotten, the sequence must be restarted. Artificial aids such as using the fingers are forbidden.

* * *

Repeat "My right arm gets heavy . . . My right arm gets heavy." Then, after a while, continue with "My left arm gets heavy and my right arm gets heavy and warm." Then "Both my arms get heavy and warm." Then, "My arms and

my right leg get heavy and warm . . . My arms and legs get heavy and warm"
. . . and eventually, "My whole body gets heavy and warm." Your arms, legs
and later your whole body really do get heavy and warm: it has been proved
by weighing test persons. This is because the blood is drained from the brain.
My psychiatrist said that mountaineers, who had practiced this exercise, had
come back from exposure to blizzards without ill effects, while other members
of the party suffered frostbite.

* * *

Hyperventilate for a few moments—deep breaths—and then hold your
breath for as long as you can. Resist the impulse to exhale. It is a real effort,
physical and psychological, taking every bit of your will and concentration. It
wipes out *all other thoughts.* When you can't hold out any longer, just e-x-h-a-
l-e blissfully and inhale a life-giving intake of air. Your mind will be "empty"
of all other thoughts. The rhythm of breathing will take over naturally. You
will be ready for sleep.

FOOD AND DRINK—AND A BIT OF POT

Take three or four drops of peppermint essence in tepid water and you will
sleep like an angel.

* * *

Before retiring, put a tablespoon of whiskey in a teacup full of hot milk. Sit
in an easy chair—no talking, reading or television—and sip it slowly, heaving
a deep sigh after each sip. Oh boy, what a lovely medicine!

* * *

Mix two teaspoonfuls of oatmeal with a little cold milk and a teaspoonful
of honey. Fill up with hot milk.

* * *

Keep a small bottle of cider and a box of fudge beside the bed to increase the blood sugar if you lie awake hungry.

* * *

Take a nightcap of whiskey every night. I've drunk four bottles a week for fifty years and it's never done me any harm.

* * *

Take an onion the size of a tennis ball and cut it into rings. Place in a jug and pour on boiling water. Let it stand for a short while, stirring occasionally. Then strain and drink warm at bedtime.

* * *

Marijuana is a great help. Since it distorts one's sense of the passage of time, it removes the feeling of guilt that comes from being awake when the rest of the world is sleeping virtuously.

BODY CULTURE

> I prepare sensibly for rest, for my sleep and dreams. I am particularly careful always to eat good food. I drink the best wine—but very little of them. I always try to be an agreeable table companion and man of the world without ever exerting myself more than is strictly necessary. After this I go to bed, well pleased with myself and others, and sleep the sleep of the just.
>
> —Brillat-Savarin

* * *

The secret of sleep is to be more physically than mentally tired. That may not be easy to calibrate, but perhaps while you are walking, jogging, cycling or skating to ensure physical readiness for sleep, you may release some of these mental tensions. If running around the block doesn't ready you for sleep, sit up in bed and roll your head as if it were a ball attached to your neck with a thread. Roll it until you hear the bones crack. Rotate your shoulders: one at a time, forward and backward and both together. Try to make your elbows meet behind you.

* * *

Dip your feet in cold water and dry them by dabbing very gently with a towel. It's important that they not be rubbed hard, since this would tend to warm them again.

* * *

I rise from my bed in the wee hours and run in place. I count a left and a right step as one count and usually go up to 475. It takes about six minutes.

* * *

If I become wide awake at night, I go into the bathroom and spend about half-an-hour reading the *Reader's Digest*, standing up throughout. I

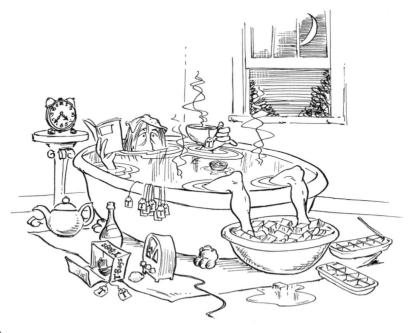

believe it reorientates the mind, and it also tires the body sufficiently to go back to sleep.

* * *

Taking a warm bath with valerian root in the water is fantastically sleep-inducing. The root can be made into a strong tea and simply poured into the tub. Or it can be suspended under the tap in a cheesecloth pouch so the water runs through it.

* * *

Take a bath in camomile tea while drinking camomile tea.

* * *

Find a friend with a soft, warm body who will hold the insomniac all night in gentle, reassuring arms.

* * *

When you can't sleep in a comfortable position, try getting into an uncomfortable position, lying flat on your face. After a few minutes of misery, turn over and enjoy the relief of being comfortable again.

ACCOUTERMENTS

I treat my insomnia with a very strong dose of camphor in my pillow and mattress.
—Van Gogh

* * *

Warmth helps the body relax, so put a woolen scarf or hood over the head —or even better, wear an old-fashioned nightcap.

* * *

Keep a clock in the bedroom. Allow a tune to enter your head and try to keep it in time with the clock's ticking.

* * *

Put three small clocks in different parts of the bedroom. Close your eyes and try to guess which tick belongs to which clock.

* * *

A hop or herb pillow helps a lot. You may be able to buy one from a health store or else you can make one yourself with a handful of kiln-dried hops put into a muslin bag.

* * *

A radio with a pillow-speaker is an invaluable aid to sleep. When you wake at an ungodly hour, you listen either to music or to chatter. Your mind is not at work reviewing situations or making plans, and in no time you are fast asleep again.

POSITIVE THINKING

Don't count sheep; talk to the shepherd.

* * *

Choose a Biblical text and deliver a sermon.

* * *

Sing in your mind.

* * *

Instead of trying desperately to get to sleep, try desperately to keep awake.

* * *

Consider getting out of bed and making a drink. If you are too tired to get out of bed, you are tired enough to go to sleep.

* * *

Stop wanting to go to sleep. At one time sleeplessness nearly drove me berserk ("How ill I shall feel tomorrow, how bad-tempered, how incapable of doing anything"), but as soon as I thought that sleep didn't really matter I began to sleep almost too much, waking as fresh as when I was a child.

* * *

When I concentrate on being glad to be alive, I soon go to sleep.

* * *

Plan to stay awake. There is nothing pleasanter after a busy day than lying in the dark, with the realization that you can enjoy the night hours without obligation to do anything.

* * *

Write a letter to the person who is most in your way. Tear it up. Write a constructive letter to an editor. Whether you mail it or not is unimportant. Something inside your head is keeping you awake. Get it on paper and "kill" it.

* * *

Whenever sleep eludes me I say to myself, "I am not allowed to sleep for another hour. I *must* keep awake." Or I pretend that it's 6:45 A.M. (my usual time for getting up is 7 o'clock), and I close my eyes "for just five minutes."

* * *

At the first hint of insomnia, I threaten myself with an hour's work. My psyche, confronted with the choice between two evils, chooses the less: I fall asleep immediately.

AND SUNDRY OTHER TIPS

If I want to sleep peacefully, I have only to take up my cards. Nothing sends me off more quickly.

—Mme. de Sévigné

* * *

Get pregnant.

* * *

Borrow my four-year-old granddaughter for a week.

* * *

Making love: the best soporific.

* * *

Making love: you don't get more sleep, but it's a hell of a lot more fun staying awake.

* * *

Read a Company Profit & Loss Statement in bed.

* * *

Force yourself to yawn and yawn.

* * *

Strictly for the clergy: I find that by preaching my last Sunday's sermon to myself, I drop off well before the end.

—Canon Peter Collins of Crayford, Kent,
in a letter to *The Times* of London

* * *

Try to recall a dream and get back into it.

* * *

Keep to a routine. Go to bed in the same way at the same time as often as you can.

or

There's no point in going to bed if you're not feeling sleepy. My regular pattern is: Monday night—awake all night reading; Tuesday—awake until about 3 A.M.; Wednesday—I sleep beautifully for about twelve hours; Thursday—awake all night; Friday—nap for about two hours at around 5 or 6 P.M., then awake until 6 A.M.; Saturday—awake all night, go to bed around 6 A.M., sleep until 3 P.M., then awake until around 3 A.M. on Monday. This method gives me enough sleep, and completely removes the anxiety about not being able to sleep.

*   *   *

I put my hand on my chest and feel my heartbeat. The rhythmic, constant beat is comforting and hypnotic. It makes me feel less alone and helps me fall asleep.

*   *   *

Find out how many hours' sleep you need on an average. Keep slightly below this so you are always sleepy when you go to bed.

*   *   *

Dogs have unspoiled natural reactions that can teach us many things. When they are ready to go to sleep they turn and turn, pulling rugs or hay or whatever is under foot into a heap, then scrunching down into it, and finally, pushing chin, jowls or ears farther down into it. When I go to bed I find that a few rudimentary turns and squirms are useful, but what seems to have an almost magical property is the pressing of my head into the pillow—a good strong push of my ear down into the "hay."

*   *   *

Repeat to yourself:

> Oh sleep! it is a gentle thing
> Beloved from pole to pole.
> To Mary Queen the praise be given!
> She sent the gentle sleep from Heaven,
> That slid into my soul.*

---

*These lines of Coleridge's were quoted to me by many correspondents as an efficacious soporific. It is probably, along with the Twenty-third Psalm, the most popular of all sleep-inducing quotations.

Yoga and the Art of Relaxation

BY NANCY PHELAN

Relaxation is, without doubt, one of the keys to sleep, but how does one set about learning the art? Many people have their own pet postures and breathing techniques, but the more I read on the subject, the more confused I become. So I decided that it would be better to offer one authoritative contribution to the subject than a dozen conflicting views. And since nearly all present-day notions about relaxation stem from one main source, Hatha Yoga, it seemed obviously sensible to invite a yoga expert to contribute to this section.

Nancy Phelan, an Australian writer, is the author of many books on different aspects of yoga, which have been translated all over the world. She is also a compulsive traveler and a distinguished writer of travel books; when you read accounts of some of the rough nights she has spent in remote and uncomfortable corners of the world, you appreciate even more the value of these relaxation techniques.

~~~~~~~~~~~~~~~~~~~~~~~~~~~~~~~~~~~~~

Though insomnia does not trouble really advanced yogis, there are a number of quite simple yoga techniques that even novices can use to help cure sleeplessness.

Before trying them, however, you should do your best to eliminate all physical contributions to insomnia. You should sleep with the window open, if practicable, but not in a draught, and your bedroom should be as dark and quiet as possible. If you live in the city and cannot escape noise, you may need to use ear-plugs or put cotton wool in your ears; and if street lights shine into your room and heavy curtains keep out too much air, you can wear a sleeping mask, or if this irritates you, put a soft scarf across your eyes.

Your mattress must not be lumpy, sagging or over-sprung, for the spine needs a solid support to rest on. When there are too many springs, the mattress gives with every movement of the body and the muscles of the back have to work all night to keep the vertebrae in position. This can hinder your sleeping, and even if you don't lie awake, you will be tired next morning. You can overcome this if you put a board under your mattress.

High pillows, which also displace the spine, can make you restless. Unless you must have one because of heart trouble, for instance, or asthma, it is best to sleep without a pillow.

If you are a bad sleeper, you should certainly not eat large, heavy meals late at night, though it is equally a mistake to go to bed hungry. You cannot expect to sleep if you go on working till all hours without giving your mind a chance to slow down before bedtime, nor if you stay up late reading or watching television when you are really ready for bed. Once the critical moment for falling asleep is lost, one gets a second wind, the brain wakes up again and eventually becomes overactive.

Probably the worst and most insidious obstacles to sleep are mental or emotional. Fruitless anger, hostility, envy, anxiety churning endlessly round in the mind build up tension till sleep becomes impossible; so does worrying about insomnia, which is one of the surest ways to prolong it.

There are two essentials for anyone who is really serious about curing insomnia through yoga: faith in the method, in yoga's power to help, and acceptance of the yoga belief that with sleep *quality* is more important than *quantity*. Once you understand this, an enormous weight is lifted from your mind, for if the quality is high enough, there is no need to sleep nine or ten hours every night. Many people doing vitally important work can function on a few hours' rest because they receive the maximum refreshment in the shortest time. And the quality of sleep can be raised through mastery of relaxation, the secret of which is correct breathing.

This method of breathing is the basis of the whole Hatha Yoga system: it is the key to discharging nervous tension (the greatest impediment to sleep), to increasing vital energy and improving general health. Yet it is not hard to learn; in fact, it is the natural respiration of animals, young babies, anyone who has not been taught wrong breathing, as so many of us were at school.

The extraordinary thing is that even mental worries and emotional distress can be lessened through yoga breathing. On the purely physical plane, as the body tempo is lowered, the mind grows calmer and quieter and bodily agitation decreases. When this form of breathing becomes part of your daily life you find a completely different attitude developing towards things you formerly thought urgent, threatening, insuperable.

Since yoga breathing is practiced standing, sitting or lying down, bad sleepers can use it in bed at night as a means of relaxing tension. You should lie flat on your back, without a pillow, with your fingertips touching, resting on your solar plexus, the area of the waistline. Breathe in slowly, through the nose, and at the same time let the abdomen come forward as though inflating yourself like a frog. The fingers should move apart. Do not raise the chest or shoulders. Continue inhaling and inflating the abdomen, gradually expanding the lower ribs, then the middle ribs and finally the top of the chest. Be sure you are expanding the chest, not heaving it up like an old-fashioned drill sergeant. You have now inhaled all the air you want and your lungs are full. To empty them, draw in the abdomen as you breathe out and continue exhaling till the lungs have been emptied. The fingertips should now be touching again.

Read this carefully several times. It may seem complicated on paper, but once you begin to draw in the breath properly you will find the whole process becomes automatic.

When it is done in bed, apart from the pacifying power of the breath, the feel of the rhythmical rise and fall of the abdomen under your fingers and the slow, quiet respiration have a soothing, almost hypnotic effect which sends many people off to sleep. But if you are a confirmed insomniac, you cannot expect to get instant results. You must persevere, practicing the slow, peaceful rhythm, with your mind concentrated on the breathing and on the knowledge that it is discharging tension, slowing down the whole body tempo, resting the heart, calming the mind and nervous system.

This complete yoga breath, which is done at a much slower rate than ordinary breathing, employs the diaphragm and full lung capacity. In everyday so-called Shallow Breathing, the diaphragm is not moved and the lungs are filled from the top, but since the breath is not a full inhalation they are never completely filled nor completely emptied; a residue of stale air remains in the lungs causing headaches, lethargy, depression, insomnia.

It is important to understand how and why the yoga breath has its effect; otherwise, you are likely to forget or make mistakes in practicing. The movement of the abdomen is essential. When it is "inflated" and brought forward, the diaphragm, the large flat muscle between chest and abdomen, is lowered and flattened. This causes a vacuum in the bottom of the lungs and the inhaled air begins to accumulate there. As the breath is continued and the chest expanded, the lungs fill completely. When the abdomen is drawn in, in exhalation, the diaphragm returns to its normal position, causing the lungs to start emptying the stale air.

All breathing is done through the nose, unless told otherwise for specific purposes. The slow rate allows adequate time for the bloodstream to take from the lungs the nourishment needed for the body cells, so the longer the inhaled air is held in the lungs the more oxygen the blood will absorb. This breathing benefits the whole system and when the general standard of health is improved, sleep also improves.

As well as taking in more oxygen with the full yoga breath, the body receives more *prana*. This Life Force or Vital Energy is in the air, as for instance vitamin D is in sunlight, and the fuller the inhalation, the more *prana* is absorbed. The pranic theory, which is the basis of all yoga breathing, can only be touched on here, but it is through complete control of *prana* that advanced yogis are able to perform extraordinary feats and live to a great age while retaining a youthful appearance.

For bad sleepers we recommend one of the *Pacifying Breathing Cycles* which you can practice by an open window before getting into bed, or indeed at any time of the day:

1. Close your eyes, and as you slowly inhale, raise the arms from the sides, cross them in front of the body, bring them up over the head and down to the sides again, describing a circle. The arms go UP with inhalation and come DOWN with exhalation. *Repeat this movement four times.*

2. Inhale, raising the arms up at the sides till the fingers touch above the head. Exhale, lowering arms to the sides. *Repeat three times.*

3. Inhale, raising arms forward and parallel till they are over the head. Exhale, lowering them. *Repeat twice.*

It is not much good doing breathing exercises before bed, then spending the night hunched up under the blankets, inhaling your own stale breath. It is better to train your body to breathe properly even while you are asleep.

During the night one lies either on the right side, the left side, on the back or on the stomach, so if the body is taught to breathe correctly, lying in these four positions while conscious, it will continue to do so whichever way one lies during the night. Once you have learnt the abdominal breath, practice it lying in the four following positions on the floor:

1. On the back.
2. On the stomach, arms by sides, face turned to one side. (If you use this position in bed, you must do so without a pillow.)
3. On the left side, with left knee drawn up and right leg stretched. Stretch the left arm above your head (along the floor) and rest your head on it. The right arm lies behind your back to ensure the chest is not restricted.
4. On the right side in exactly the same position in reverse.

These poses are also excellent for relaxing. Naturally, you would not sleep with your head resting on your arm all night but the position is comfortable when lying on the floor.

Once you know how to breathe correctly, you can begin learning how to relax at will. *Savasana* (Corpse Pose or Pose of Complete Rest) is a yoga *asana* (bodily position) which, when done properly, relaxes every muscle in turn, discharges nervous tension, empties the mind and recharges the system with fresh vitality. It has been used and adapted in various forms by many healers, even beauty experts, and it is a powerful remedy for fatigue, as well as for nervous, physical, and mental tension. It is both simple and difficult . . . simple to try and difficult to master, yet anyone can learn it with patience and perseverance.

Savasana is usually practiced on the floor but you can also do it in bed.

Lie on your back, without a pillow, and close your eyes. Your arms should be by your sides with your hands limp, with open palms, and your legs and feet together.

Slow down your respiration and concentrate for a few minutes on yoga breathing to help calm your mind and make it more receptive; then begin to relax the muscles, starting with the tips of the toes and working slowly up through the whole body, taking each part in turn: feet, ankles, calves, knees; thighs, hips, stomach muscles, the small of the back. Relax the chest and shoulders, the arms and hands and fingers. Relax the neck and face muscles. Let the lower jaw sag, the tongue go limp, turn your eyes back under the lids. Smooth out the forehead . . . no frowning, no tension between the eyebrows. Maintain the slow breathing all the time.

Check through your body to see you haven't missed any part, and if you find muscular tension—perhaps in the jaw or in the small of the back—persuade it to let go, gently, gradually. Forcing or trying too hard to relax usually causes more tension.

With your muscles relaxed and slow, steady yoga breathing established, imagine that you are letting go completely, mentally and physically. You don't need to hold on any more; you are sinking down into the darkness, almost down through the floor, as you sometimes feel before falling asleep. Think of the tide going out, draining away from the shore, and try to let yourself go with it. Imagine the nervous energy draining out of your system, leaving your body heavy and lifeless, unable to lift a finger. Nothing matters. You don't have to worry. All the messages from the brain have ceased; you are at peace.

All the time you are maintaining your deep, slow yoga breathing, letting the abdomen come forward with inhalation and fall back with exhalation. The peaceful rhythm, the slower tempo are calming your whole mind and body, relaxing your nerves, discharging tension and at the same time supplying your system with *prana* or vital energy, which is food for the nerves.

Now escape completely. Leave your body lying on the floor and get away from your room, your present life, your work, family, worries, responsibilities. Transport yourself to some peaceful place that you know or that you have created in your mind . . . a personal hermitage where you can retreat whenever you want and from whence you can return each time refreshed. Make sure it is a complete escape, that you leave everything behind. Your problems will still be there when you come back, but you will have more strength to cope with them.

Now, switch off all thoughts and pictures and try to keep your mind empty. Try to see nothing, to think of nothing. Turn your eyes up under the closed lids; it helps to empty the mind. Continue your slow, rhythmical breathing.

When *Savasana* is done during the day, you then stretch, yawn and open your eyes, but if done in bed, for insomnia, it is better to remain just as you are but to stop trying to keep the mind blank, which you might find taking too much effort if you go on too long. When you have really achieved emptiness of mind you have reached the beginning of complete relaxation and will "come back," as it were, from ten minutes of *Savasana* more refreshed than from eight hours of sleep.

Traditionally yoga is always learnt from a teacher; even in the West, when *Savasana* is taught, the pupil is instructed in each stage of relaxation by the teacher, always in a slow, quiet voice. However, many students learn to "switch on" this voice in the mind like a tape or record, for practising at home. Perhaps you could get someone to read the instructions to you after you are in bed, or if you have a tape recorder, read them yourself onto a tape and use it when you want it. Be sure to speak slowly, leaving long pauses between each phrase. Part of the technique is the sameness, the repetitive quality of the monologue.

As well as deep breathing, breathing cycles and *Savasana*, there are several simple forms of Spinal Massage which have a soothing effect on the nervous system and will help you to sleep if you do them just before bedtime. They massage the spinal column and the roots of the spinal nerves.

1. Sit on the floor with legs stretched and together, and your hands under your thighs. Keeping your legs straight, roll back and bring them right over the

head till your toes touch the floor, then come up and forward till your head touches your knees, if possible.

Roll back again, then forward again, slowly and carefully, turning yourself into a rocking chair, and keeping the movement smooth and rhythmical.

Repeat three or four times, but be sure that you are putting pressure on your spine, not rolling over to one side, or the effect will be lost.

Now, cross your legs at the ankles, take hold of your toes and continue the rocking movement . . . back to touch the floor with your toes above your head, if you can, then right forward again; then back, then forward, until pleasantly tired. Never force or strain yourself.

2. This second Spinal Massage is very easy, pleasant and soothing.

Lie on your back on the floor, draw your knees up to the body and cross your ankles. Clasp your arms round your legs so they are held close to you, shut your eyes and gently rock from side to side, as though in a cradle, massaging the spine and the roots of the spinal nerves.

If you feel you would like to try a more advanced yoga *asana* which has direct healing effects on insomnia, you must first make sure you have no serious spinal condition such as easily displaced discs or deterioration of the neck vertebrae.

The *Pose of Tranquillity* is rather difficult for anyone not used to yoga practice and demands balance and control, but it is an extremely important method of inducing tranquillity and sleep. It puts pressure on a nerve centre at the back of the head which is closely connected with the power of sleeping. Many people have freed themselves from taking sleeping pills through regular practice of this pose.

Lie down on the floor on your back. Raise your arms over your head (along the floor).

Try to bring your legs up and over your body, keeping them straight, until they are above you at an angle of 45 degrees. Then raise the arms, keeping them straight, and let the legs rest on the palms. The area of contact for most people is round about the kneecaps but it varies, since everyone has different proportions. You have to find your own position for yourself, and you will know when you have it because you feel perfectly comfortable and secure. This pose is held by *balance* and unless the balance is right you will not get the benefits. These come from the pressure put on a nerve centre at the back of the head which affects the power of sleep, and the pressure is only effective when the body is in the correct position.

Body, arms and legs form a triangle. The legs *rest* on the open palms; there should be no need to hold on with the hands if the balance is correct. (Arms and legs must be kept *straight*, to balance.) Shut your eyes, inhale and exhale the full yoga breath and focus your mind on peace. Hold the pose as long as is comfortable, the longer the better.

To complete the *asana*, bring the legs down over the head, split them apart, bend the knees and take hold of them with your hands, pressing them to the floor, one on each side of the head. Then let go and slowly lower arms and legs to the floor.

With the exception of the *Pose of Tranquillity*, which should be attempted with caution, all these simple methods may be safely practiced by anyone, and if done properly and systematically, will help to defeat insomnia. They may also serve as a first step in learning more about this remarkable system and philosophy which have helped so many people all over the world.

Gadgets and Gimmicks, Fads and Fancies

Perhaps calling this section on sleep aids by a flippant title is unfair to the manufacturers of all the sleep merchandise on the market—from a glamorous sleep mask "in an alluring leopard print sateen," through bed socks, magnetic pillows and anti-snore balls, to highly sophisticated electronic apparatus. There are people who have sleep problems, and there are also sleep buffs who pursue the perfect night's rest with a zeal that borders on fanaticism. On the whole, the sleep shops and the mail-order sleep business cater to the latter. I can't pretend to feel much enthusiasm for most of this stuff. But if, as I'm sure is the case, the goods described on the following pages have all been tried and tested and proved efficacious, has one the right to scoff?

By the same token, I may be thought unsympathetic by those readers who are deeply attached to their sleep-time rituals, however eccentric, or as with tea and coffee addicts, downright illogical. There are some, for instance, who put their

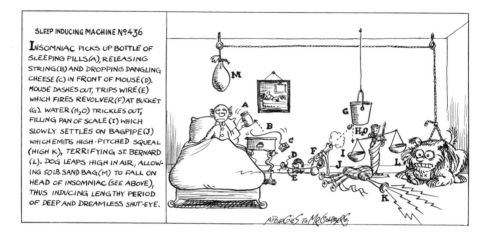

SLEEP INDUCING MACHINE Nº 436

INSOMNIAC PICKS UP BOTTLE OF SLEEPING PILLS (A), RELEASING STRING (B) AND DROPPING DANGLING CHEESE (C) IN FRONT OF MOUSE (D). MOUSE DASHES OUT, TRIPS WIRE (E) WHICH FIRES REVOLVER (F) AT BUCKET (G). WATER (H_2O) TRICKLES OUT, FILLING PAN OF SCALE (I) WHICH SLOWLY SETTLES ON BAGPIPE (J) WHICH EMITS HIGH-PITCHED SQUEAL (HIGH K), TERRIFYING ST. BERNARD (L). DOG LEAPS HIGH IN AIR, ALLOWING 50 LB. SAND BAG (M) TO FALL ON HEAD OF INSOMNIAC (SEE ABOVE), THUS INDUCING LENGTHY PERIOD OF DEEP AND DREAMLESS SHUT-EYE.

APOLOGIES TO MR. GOLDBERG.

faith in hot baths as a somnifacient; others claim hot baths keep them awake and prefer cold ones, and a Spartan rubdown with a coarse towel. Then there are those who trust in exercise or in sex as their own reliable soporific. Who is to say which have the right answers? I do not wish to disparage any individual's personal or idiosyncratic solutions, but in this whole contentious area I find myself ultimately in agreement with Arnold Bennett, himself a long-suffering victim of sleeplessness, when he wrote:

> I doubt if there is any remedy for insomnia considered as insomnia. Sleeplessness is a symptom of disease, not the disease itself. It can only be cured indirectly and by specialized professional skill. Few bad sleepers realise this. Just as a man with a weak heart will marvellously abstain from learning about that organ, so will the bad sleeper continue to sleep badly for decades without seriously inquiring into the root of the evil or causing it to be inquired into.

> Palliatives of the symptom exist: monotonous repetitions, keeping the mind empty, food, warm drink, cool drink, warm bath, cold bath, physical exercise to restore the circulation of the blood, etc., etc. And some of them are sometimes temporarily effective. But none of them will cure the ailment of which insomnia

is a symptom. All of them are in conception unscientific, empiric, quack, and come under the sinister classification of "muddling through." The idea of "inducing sleep" is absurd. Sleep ought not to have to be enticed like a frightened fawn. It should pounce on you like a tiger.

〜〜〜〜〜〜〜〜〜〜〜〜〜〜〜〜〜〜〜〜

THE HYPNOTIC WAY

Of all the domestic mechanical aids to sleep I investigated, one seemed to stand out as being simpler, cheaper and more effective than the others—the autohypnotic cassette. The hypnotic trance is not in itself real sleep; breathing, muscle reflexes and the flow of blood to the brain continue the same in the waking state or in trance. But hypnotism can be helpful in overcoming insomnia. It certainly is not effective in every case. It isn't likely to work, for instance, with the severely depressed or the psychotic, and some individuals have such a powerful built-in resistance to hypnotism that no hypnotic art is likely to prevail with them. But those who are desperate for want of sleep are likely to be more susceptible subjects than most. If the hypnotherapist asks for their trust and promises them the sleep they crave, they have little to lose and much to gain.

Obviously, few people can afford the fees of a hypnotist for a session in their own home, and you can't expect to have a nighttime's rest induced in a doctor's consulting room. Here is where the hypnotic tape comes in. You can dispense with the traditional hand movements made in front of your eyes, but you do need the persuasive voice telling you that you are getting drowsier and drowsier. The presence of the recorded voice in your bedroom isn't simply a solace to the lonely, it also serves to silence what for many is the greatest enemy of sleep —that internal phonograph record forever stuck in the groove of recrimination or self-reproach.

What sort of message is put over on these tapes? I tried out one now on the market* which had been strongly recommended by a number of insomniac victims, and subsequently obtained a transcript from the psychotherapist who had devised it.

The cassette has two sides. The purpose of the first, which you are asked to listen to at any time before going to bed, is to instill confidence that the cassette is going to work. So it begins on a strongly positive note:

> Every day perhaps a dozen people come into my consulting room and say, "Doctor, please let me have some sleeping tablets." Of each of these people I ask three questions: Are you in pain? Is it noisy? Or are you worried about something? In most cases it's worry. But regardless of the reason why you can't sleep, what you are going to learn now is going to help you get rid of your insomnia once and for all.

> The strange thing about insomnia is that although nearly everyone suffers from it at one time or another, it isn't a disease. It isn't even a very interesting mental condition and it isn't in the least bit difficult to cure! If you don't believe that, you are going to have a surprise in store for you this evening. If you want to, tonight and every night from now on, you are going to be able to sleep naturally and soundly.

After this encouraging start the speaker, who has a deep, avuncular but quite sexy voice, goes on to give a simple explanation of the mechanics of sleep and to explode various myths about sleep requirements—that everyone needs eight hours' sleep a night, for instance, or that we should all be expected to rise bright and cheerful at dawn each morning:

> The way things are set up in our society, everyone is supposed to be in bed around ten or eleven at night and up again at around six or seven. From the time you get

*Therapy Tapes, Northmead, Ribblesdale Avenue, Clitheroe, Lancashire, England.

up in the morning to the time you go to bed, you are supposed to be bright and alert. If you doze off for a few minutes in the middle of the day, people look at you as though there was something wrong. "Did you have a late night?" they ask, or "Aren't you feeling well?" Now, the strange thing is that many people function much better on two or even three short naps than on a single period of sleep. In some countries they recognise this and you find the idea of the siesta widely accepted. A lot of people find it difficult to stay asleep for more than three or four hours at a time. If you are one of them and if you find yourself wanting to doze off during the middle of the day after a short night's sleep, it is very likely that you are one of the many people who need a different sleep pattern from the one that our society seems to think we ought to have. The sooner we all realise that each one of us is an individual with our own individual requirements, the sooner we will all stop feeling that being different is somehow the same as being wrong.

Good stuff, in my view, and I also liked the passage about sleeping pills:

And now I want you to make a decision. If you're suffering from insomnia, the chances are that you are taking sleeping tablets or sedatives of some sort of other. If you listen to the other side of this recording and if you decide you want to cure your insomnia, then you'll never need to take another sleeping tablet or sedative in your life. I ought to ask you to take those pills and throw them away. The best thing to do would be to flush them down the drain. I should ask you to do this here and now because I want to prove to you right from the very beginning that you don't need them, and to prove to yourself you don't want to need them. How about putting them somewhere out of reach, say just for a couple of days; then when you look at them and wonder why you ever bothered with such things, you can throw them away.

The first side ends by asking you to practice switching off the machine in the dark, as the second side is to be listened to only when you are already in bed with the lights off.

On the second side, you are instructed in a slow, increasingly drawling voice, to relax each part of your body in turn, starting with the feet and working up to the head. It is, in fact, a very simple version of the yoga technique of *Savasana* (see previous chapter), plus repeated assertions that you are getting sleepier and sleepier. It must surely rank as one of the most boring tapes ever recorded. I wasn't surprised when the psychotherapist who made it told me that the recording session for side 2 took sixteen hours because the sound engineer, like Alice's Dormouse, repeatedly fell asleep; and he himself had only managed to keep awake by taking a triple dose of amphetamines. I am convinced that it works for many chronic insomniacs, too, because it's so boring to listen to that you'd rather go to sleep than have to hear it for a second time.

PERFECTION IN PILLOWS

Perhaps you have managed all these years with one standard-size down or foam pillow from your local department store, but some people care passionately about the number and shape and filling of their pillows. Here is how Charles P. Kelly, author of *The Natural Way to Healthful Sleep* and a sleep buff *par excellence*, describes his solution to the perennial problem of how many, which and where:

> To maintain a normal position of the head and neck during sleep, the present writer uses three pillows, two rather soft and flat, the third flat but very firm. When sleeping on his back, one soft pillow is used. On his side, a soft pillow is used on top of the firm one, the two raising his head enough above the mattress to keep his neck in line with his spine. The advantage of the two pillows over one large soft one is that sufficient height is secured without having the head sink deeply into the pillow, which would cause overheating and make a change of position more difficult. A dislocation of his right shoulder several years ago which was diagnosed and treated as rheumatism left that shoulder so sensitive to pressure that sleeping on his right side is not possible. With the double pillow near one side of the bed and the single soft one adjoining it, shifting to the low pillow when

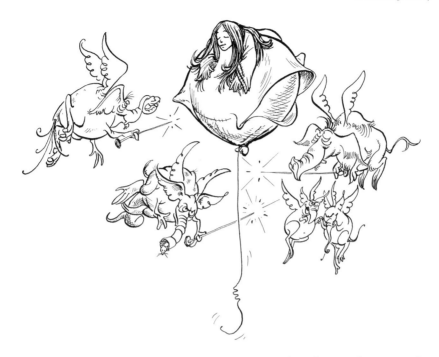

turning to the back position is so easy that it is often done without complete awakening.

Recently after sleeping two or three months on a new and firmer mattress, mostly on his left side, the author began to have pains in his left shoulder, such as ordinarily can be attributed to arthritis or bursitis. Suspecting that the pains might be due simply to too much pressure of the shoulder against the new firm mattress, a pad about twelve by eighteen inches was placed under his body just below the armpit, in this way taking his body's weight off the painful shoulder. Without further treatment the pains disappeared within a few days and have not returned. The pad used was made by folding a cotton blanket and covering it with a small pillowcase. Naturally after this experience the pad was not discarded but was kept as a permanent part of the bed's equipment, just as the head pillows are.

With the use of this underarm pad the left side position became so entirely comfortable that the back position was used very little. The result was that after a short time twinges of pain began to occur in the upper shoulder, the right one, which had been made sensitive by a previous injury. The right arm had been allowed to rest on the mattress in front of the body, and upon consideration it seemed likely that the weight of the arm had pulled the shoulder joint down into an irritating position. A plump pillow was then placed on the mattress in front of the body so that it would hold the right forearm almost level with the shoulder. The pains disappeared promptly and have not returned. This pillow, too, has been retained in permanent use.

Wuensch's store in East Orange, New Jersey, which inherited the Sleep Center business of the famous Norman Dine of New York (dubbed "Public Sandman" by *The New Yorker* and "the Dean of Beducation" by *Time* magazine), has at least twelve different kinds of pillows for the Kellys of this world —though to be fair to Kelly, he believes in do-it-yourself pillow making, and his book describes ways you yourself can soften or harden or thicken or thin the store-bought article. But if you want the perfect pillow without involving yourself with ticking and polystyrene, Wuensch's will sell you, *inter alia*, a Stay Plump Pillow, a Contour Pillow, an Angulation Pillow, a Virile Pillow (for "the full-sized man"), an inflatable Cradle-Air Travel Pillow that fits one's purse, and —my own personal favorite—a pillow that conceals a small speaker and comes complete with long cord and plug so that you can tune your pillow into a radio, TV set or recordplayer (mono or stereo) and listen peacefully without disturbing your neighbor.

Elsewhere you can buy He and She Pillows, the former being made of goose feathers, the latter of down. The theory is that you should choose your filling according to the pressure your head exerts on the pillow; a man's head tends to be three pounds heavier than a woman's—10 lbs. against 7 lbs. on an average. Or if you dislike soft pillows, you can invest in a traditional Japanese wooden pillow, like a little footstool on short legs, designed to fit only the neck so as not to disturb elaborate Japanese hairdos.

Many of the pillows I've described will sell well without benefit of medical endorsement. But a number of hard-sell pillow manufacturers have marketed their product with the backing of medical experts. Reading these blurbs, you start to wonder how you ever managed to sleep on the common-or-garden-variety pillow or what fearful risks you ran with your health. Here, for instance, is the text of a leaflet exhorting you to buy a Posture Pillow:

Why You Should Sleep on a Posture Pillow

The skeleton of the human neck consists of seven bones or vertebrae, which are responsible for holding the head in a correct postural position on the shoulders, carrying the arteries to the brain, and protecting the delicate spinal cord. (It has exactly the same number of vertebrae as a giraffe or a swan.)

This vital structure is well able to do its job whilst one is in an upright position, but an abnormal and excessive strain is placed on it when lying down. This is caused by the incorrect support provided by conventionally shaped pillows.

The standard flat pillow tends to push the head either too far forward or to one side, throwing strain upon the vertebrae, the discs which separate them (which act as shock absorbers), and the supporting ligaments and muscles. This can cause, or aggravate, such conditions as: arthritis, spondylosis, slipped disc, painful or stiff muscles and ligaments, and headache.

The Posture Pillowcase was designed by a leading London Orthopaedic Specialist to convert a normal feather pillow into the "butterfly" shape recommended by Physiotherapists. It has a narrow central waist which balances and supports the head and neck in the correct anatomical position, whilst the butterfly wings help to maintain this during sleep.

Some people put their faith in magnetic pillows. At Bell and Croydon in London you can buy a Slumber Aid Pillow, which has eight thin, flexible static magnets placed between two sheets of very soft foam plastic—"each magnet magnetised in a special way to produce a continuous field without the use of batteries or other power." How does it work? According to the publicity handout,

> It has been scientifically established that the brain operates with minute electrical impulses. Our research and field testing have led us to believe that the magnets in your Slumber Aid will send out minute impulses which will be picked up by the brain. After a few nights, an affinity is built up between the Slumber Aid and the brain, thus reducing tension and inducing sleep. A high degree of effectiveness has been shown in our tests, and in most cases sleep has improved. Owing to its gentle nature, it may take a few days before you derive benefit from its use, but PERSIST with it. This is most important.

It may be no reflection on Bell and Croydon or the manufacturers of the Slumber Aid Pillow, but The British Medical Association is not able to endorse these sleep aids. Their pamphlet *Sleeping and Not Sleeping*, by Ian Oswald, says tersely: "Magnetic pillows are a waste of money."

NOSTRUMS FOR NOISE

Noise is certainly a major obstacle to sleep, particularly sudden loud noise like the passing of heavy trucks or low-flying aircraft. Some people can sleep through the loudest clash and clatter, others need the protection of heavy curtains, double glazing and other sound-insulation devices. If these don't solve your problem, you will probably need earplugs. One sleep shop, selling earplugs of soft plastic, "scientifically pre-shaped," urges you to buy three pairs—small, medium and large—to make sure you have a perfect fit.

But if you want to save your money, you can always make your own. Here is the advice of the indefatigable Charles P. Kelly:

A durable and very effective earplug can easily be made from a pencil-cap eraser. It should be of soft rubber and of a size to fit the ear. With a sharp knife or a razor blade, moistened, the solid part of the eraser is trimmed away until only the cup remains. Sharp corners are smoothed with a fine file or sandpaper. A dozen or so strands of wool crochet yarn are tied round with spool thread. With a thin sliver of wood or metal resting on this tie, the strands of yarn are forced into the rubber cup. Scissors are used to trim the ends of the yarn flush with the rubber. There should be enough strands of yarn to fit moderately tight in the rubber cup, but not enough to bulge it. Holding the cup by the closed end, the open end is moistened slightly in the mouth and then forced firmly into the ear. A very small perforation in the bottom of the cup will ensure against uncomfortable air pressure in the ear. A pair of these plugs well fitted will materially dull the hearing and bring extra hours of sleep.

Mr. Kelly also has a neat and logical way of dealing with intermittent noises. He suggests drowning them with a continuous noise:

An electric fan can be used to produce a continuous noise, even when it is not needed for cooling. If its noise is not loud enough, it can be placed on a wood or metal support which will act as a sounding board. Removing felt or rubber pads under the fan base will make it still louder. To prevent the fan from "walking" off its support, cut surgeon's adhesive tape in lengths three times its width, fold these lengths into squares with the gum outward, and apply them under the fan's base. Placing the support of the fan in contact with the bedstead will make its noise seem still louder.

SLEEP SUNDRIES

New electronic gadgets for the insomniac appear on the market as frequently as new kinds of sleeping pills, and perhaps for the same reason: the beneficial effect of any sleep aid, however trusted, is likely to pall after a while if the underlying cause of the insomnia still exists.

Take your pick. There's a Magic Finger Bed Massager, for instance, which comes complete with automatic timer. You can attach it yourself without special tools, they say, in ten minutes, and it gives thirty minutes of massage. "You go to sleep with massage and you wake up with massage," runs the blurb —provided, I suppose, that you take care to wake up within the half-hour. An English equivalent is the Sleeptite. This consists of two solid plastic shapes— one like an inverted top hat contains the motor which produces sleep-inducing vibrations. This is hooked securely to the bedsprings. The second, smaller shape goes on the bedside table and is attached to the first by a long electric wire. When you want to drop off, you press the knob on top and the "vibrator" produces a sort of "muffled motion-cum-sound." "A clatter of wheels" comes through the pillows and the bed pulsates. The motor turns itself off after fifteen minutes.

Or how about a brain-lulling Sleep Conditioner, which emits a "drowsing sound" to tranquilize the overactive mind or to screen off disturbing noises from the outside? (Mr. Kelly would say that a common electric fan would do as well.) Another machine produces a continuous waterfall sound known as "white noise."

If you prefer not to use up the earth's dwindling energy resources, there are plenty of nonelectronic sleep aids on the market. For a start, there is all the special apparel. Simulated hand-knit socks for the chilly feet are available, or a sleeping cap with an adjustable chin band for the sparsely thatched pate. For the snorer, there's the Anti-Snore Ball which attaches to a man's pajamas and discourages him from turning over on his back, the posture most likely to produce the snore; or a special elasticized chin mask to make sure he (it's mostly he, it seems) keeps his mouth shut all night. There are masks galore, including a de luxe mask in treated satin for the creamed face, with room for the lashes to move freely. And if you can't sleep and feel like a smoke in bed, there's a Robot Cigarette Holder. You puff serenely through a cooling long tube, and an adjustable holder grips the cigarette to ensure that the ash falls safely into a chrome tray. You can buy a single tube alone or a Dual Model, which allows both partners to smoke at the same time.

There is also a wide assortment of herbal products. These have a long tradition of efficacy. In 1801, we read, "His Majesty George III received more benefit in his late illness from a hop pillow than from the stronger narcotics." Jacksons of Piccadilly sells a potpourri of Sleep Herbs, and very odoriferous it is: I tried it out recently when my pajamas had an unfortunate encounter with some pickled herring in an overnight bag. Sleep herbs won. Then there are special bath salts. You can put a tablespoon of a tranquilizing balsam essence into your bath. "Immerse yourself for twenty tension-easing minutes; pat yourself dry—no rubbing. Slip into bed! Sleep better or money refunded."

Ogden Nash deserves the last word on Sleep Sundries:

WHAT, NO SHEEP

WHAT, NO SHEEP? These are a few of the 600 products sold in the "sleep shop" of a New York department store.

—From an advertisement of the Consolidated Edison Company in the New York Times.

I don't need no sleepin' medicine—
I seen a ad by ole Con Edison.
Now when I lay me on my mattress
You kin hear me snore from Hell to Hatteras,
With muh Sleep Record,
Muh Vaporizer,
Muh Electric Slippers,
Muh Yawn Plaque,
Muh Slumber Buzzer,
Muh miniature Electric Organ,
An' muh wonderful Electric Blanket.

My old woman couldn't eat her hominy—
Too wore out from the durned insominy.
She give insominy quite a larrupin',
Sleeps like a hibernatin' tarrapin,
With her Eye Shade,
Her Clock Radio,
Her Sinus Mask,
Her Massagin' Pillow,
Her Snore Ball,
Her miniature Electric Organ,
An' her Wonderful Electric Blanket.

Evenin's when the sunlight westers
I pity muh pioneer an-cestors.
They rode the wilderness wide and high,
But how did they ever go sleepy-bye
Without their Eye Shade,
Their Clock Radio,
Their Sleep Record,
Their Vaporizer,
Their Sinus Mask,
Their Electric Slippers,
Their Yawn Plaque,
Their Slumber Buzzer,
Their Massagin' Pillow,
Their Snore Ball,
Their miniature Electric Organ,
An' their wonderful Electric Blanket?

NIGHTCAPS

Whenever two or three obsessional insomniacs are gathered together—which,
on the law of averages, must happen with growing frequency these days—the
conversation will often turn to the relative virtues of different kinds of night-

caps, and particularly to the pros and cons of tea and coffee, or a glass of Scotch.

The tea/coffee dispute can wage quite fiercely at times, and there are obviously strong cultural reasons for some people preferring one beverage and some the other. A friend told me recently how astonished a French waiter was, busy serving late-night black coffee to his compatriots, when an English couple ordered tea. "How can they hope to sleep?" he demanded. But the fact is that both tea and coffee (and Coca-Cola, for that matter) contain caffeine, which is one of the psychotropic drugs (drugs which act on the central nervous system) classified as stimulants. Amphetamines come under the same classification. Both drugs decrease fatigue and increase mental and physical activity. The effects of caffeine have been studied in some detail: small doses (between 65 and 130 milligrams) may not affect you, but the more you take, the more certain it is that both the quality and the duration of your sleep will be impaired, and this will be true regardless of your age, sex or previous addiction to caffeine. Not everyone will be equally affected: genetic factors certainly play a role in drug response, and account for individual differences in drug tolerance or speed of reaction. But it is clear that on the whole, tea and coffee, except in small doses, are not to be recommended to those with sleep problems. (Decaffeinated coffee is of course quite neutral in its effect. And so, no doubt, if anyone were to invent it, would be decaffeinated tea.)

Alcohol is another matter. It is classed as a depressant, and its general effect is to slow down mental processes. But it seems, nevertheless, to affect people in a variety of ways: some, perhaps most, are made drowsy after a few drinks, but others will become nervous, excitable, even bellicose. Heredity may have something to do with these different responses. We can't be sure, for the science of human pharmacogenetics, as it is called, is still only in its infancy. But there is one important effect of alcohol which should be mentioned in the nightcap context: the fact that it tends to suppress REM. The more you drink, the greater will be the effect on your dreaming. If you go to bed in a drunken stupor, you are certain to suffer some disturbance of your normal sleep pattern.

So if you are interested in alcohol as a nightcap, you must take it in moderation: just enough to make you drowsy, not enough to seriously distort your sleep and dreaming.

Some people worry about taking alcohol as a nightcap, fearing that an adequate sleep-inducing measure this week will have to be doubled next week to achieve the same effect. There may be something in this argument: in general, the human body tends to acquire tolerance for any regularly taken drug within about two weeks. So if you depend on whiskey to send you off, you could find yourself on the way to a serious alcohol problem. On the other hand, the subject of alcohol addiction is a minefield of controversy: it really requires a book in itself to sort out all the issues.

As mentioned on page 49, an ideal nightcap would seem to be milk or hot chocolate, since milk contains the amino acid called tryptophan which has been shown to possess a mild, natural, sedative effect. At one experiment at the University of Oklahoma Medical School, tryptophan was given to a group of people over a period of several weeks. The results were impressive: the volunteers fell asleep unusually quickly, awakened less during sleep and spent more time than normal in delta sleep. So the claims made for brand products with a milk basis, like Horlick's and Ovaltine, that they promote sound sleep, have a proven scientific foundation. Alas, maybe because of weaning traumas, not all of us can stomach milk at bedtime, not even for the sake of a good night's sleep.

AND SO TO BEDS

There is not in my opinion anything in nature which is more immediately calculated totally to subject health, strength, love, esteem, and indeed everything that is desirable in the married state, than that odious, most indelicate, and most hurtful custom of man and wife continually *pigging* together, in one and the same bed. Nothing more unwise—nothing more indecent—nothing more unnatural, than for a man and a woman to sleep, and snore, and steam, and do everything else that's indelicate together, three hundred and sixty-five times—every year.

The author of these remarkably vehement words was a certain Dr. James Graham who began a smart and successful practice near St. James's Palace in London in 1775. You might think that he was a Puritan, but you'd be wrong. In his youth, he had studied the new science of electricity in Philadelphia and had become fired with the notion that the pleasures of the marriage union might be intensified if it was performed under the "glowing, accelerating and most genial influences of the heaven-born, all-animating element or principle, the electrical or concocted fire!" To this end, he had constructed a "Celestial Bed" at the cost of £18,000 (a stupefying price even by today's standards). It was intricately carved and covered by the most costly silk damasks, scented by Arabian spices and it swung rhythmically with the movement of its occupants. Its most important feature was its electrification: it was mounted on six massive glass pillars and charged with electric currents. A keen lecturer and pamphleteer, Dr. Graham would invite those of his audience and readers who wished to sleep in the Celestial Bed to write for appointments "accompanied by a complement of a £50 bank note." It was apparently a wild success—despite many angry critics (Dr. Southey in his *Commonplace Book* called the bed "the infamous pandarism of a scoundrel").

The history of beds is rich with eccentric fads and notions. A man from San Francisco is said to have spent half an hour in his wife's room each night but could only fall asleep in an open coffin, which he kept obligingly in an adjoining room. Benjamin Franklin, who believed that heat was inimical to sleep, kept two beds in his freezing-cold bedroom and would move to the second bed as soon as the first became warm. Churchill was another who favored twin beds for the pleasure of moving to a fresh, unwrinkled bed halfway through the night.

Boswell mentions a certain Lord Monboddo, who woke every morning at four "and would walk naked in his room with the window open"; this he called taking an air bath, after which he went to sleep again. Johnson observed: "I suppose, Sir, there is no more in it than this: he wakes at four and cannot sleep till he chills himself and makes the warmth of the bed a grateful sensation."

The positioning of beds in the room is itself a controversial issue. Charles Dickens was in the habit of carrying a pocket compass on his travels to make sure that his bed was aligned due north and south, believing that certain magnetic currents flowed between the poles and would benefit the sleeper if it flowed in a straight line through the body. But Dickens was not an isolated eccentric in this matter; practitioners of Hatha Yoga also attach importance to this question of alignment. And that great crusader for birth control, Marie Stopes, in her idiosyncratic book *Sleep* makes a great issue of this point:

> Beds are generally placed to suit the build of the room, but this is often wrong. The place of the bed should be determined by something more fundamentally important, that is the direction of the North. The head of the bed should be north or south, and the bed should extend between these two poles. It is comparatively unimportant whether the head or the feet are at the north end of the bed, but it is very important indeed that the extension of the body should lie along a line either south-north or north-south. Few people are now aware that we do not have only five senses, as children are senselessly taught in school, but we used to have, and some few people still have, other senses, and one of these is a sense of the north. It is just as clear and definite a sense as any other. One *sees* the wall in front of one, one *hears* the bird calling, and one *magnetates* the north. Magnetates? A new word, you say. Yes. A new word, and I am coining it here and now for a very real sense. I know about it, for I possess it. It is in my spine that I magnetate the north, between my shoulder-blades and hips. I used to have this sense so intensely that I could be blind-folded in a fog on a desolate moor and twisted round a great number of times, and could at once point to the exact north. This was tested by geologists with a compass and was often of great use to me. Since my back was broken and my abdominal walls cut, I am not so acutely sensitive to the north as I was, but still I generally feel it. If by chance I visit a

house where my bed is set east-west, even though there may be nothing in the curtained room to indicate this, once I lie in the bed trying to sleep, I very soon suffer and so find out. I do not sleep till I have popped out of bed and shifted it to the north and south direction. If it is too heavy for me, I lie diametrically or slantwise across it till I am north and south, and even though this may make the bedclothes rather uncomfortable, I am then able to sleep.

There are many, certainly the majority of ordinary people and also most medical doctors, who will scoff at the idea that the north and south placing of any bed is important. That does not show that they are wise, or right, or "scientific"; it merely proves that they are ignorant of one of the existing human faculties. Many people who are quite unconscious of the faculty have a disturbed feeling which appears unaccountable when their beds are wrongly placed. I think this is because they feel subconsciously what some feel consciously.

Marie Stopes is, it must be admitted, the most intemperate dogmatist on any and every subject connected with beds and bedding. She agrees wholeheartedly with Dr. Graham, for instance, on the subject of men and women sleeping apart:

> The best way for the majority is for the wife to have a room with a double bed and the husband to have a room to himself for general use, keeping the wife's bedroom a romantic place. The "double-bedded room" is to be execrated. The miserable little shanties that are being built now instead of the comfortable houses of our forefathers are forcing the twin-bed room on people who are willing or have to put up with them. Yet many of these inhabitants get devitalised, irritable, sleepless and unhappy, I think, because of them. The twin bed set was an invention of the Devil, jealous of married bliss.

She is equally opposed to hot-water bottles "rubber, earthenware or (oh, horror!) aluminum." She regards pajamas as "the most uncomfortable sleeping garment ever devised," and is heated in her endorsement of pure-silkworm silk nightgowns ("It is iniquitous that cellulose fabrications should be allowed to call themselves 'pure silk' and so deceive women into thinking they are getting silk when they are not"). And she reserves particular indignation for soft-foam-rubber mattresses, which she says are

> an example of a modern "advance" to be avoided by all who value their health. It is pernicious. Do *not* use any rubber mattress, and do not have rubber-tyred wheels on your bedstead. Why? Because rubber is an insulator and cuts you off from electric currents of the earth with which you should be in contact. Many, sadly many, people are insulating themselves incessantly. Rubber-soled shoes all day, and then rubber covering to their floors, small wheels with rubber tyres on their beds—alas, poor things, they are being devitalised. No wonder millions at the end of the day feel limp and exhausted, yet neither ready for or able to sleep.

After the furies of Miss Stopes's prose, it is a relief to turn to the blander style of the bed manufacturers, offering the affluent bed buyer a bewildering choice of shapes and sizes: round beds, oval beds, heart-shaped beds, hanging beds, waterbeds, beds in black hide from Heals, London, at £815, or the Cadillac model of the Push Button Heaven bed from Wuensch's, offering 1,001 blissful positions with hydraulic-powered motor from $359 to $679. Wuensch's also have a Push Button bed for the thrifty—40 positions for only $99.50.

Waterbeds deserve perhaps special treatment if only because of their alleged sleep-wooing properties. I thought waterbeds were a strictly contemporary adornment to elegant living, but I discovered to my surprise that a Water Mattress was being advertised in *The Times* of London in 1854:

> HOOPER'S WATER MATTRESSES, for Bedsores, whether threatened with sloughing, or in which sloughing has actually taken place. Fractures, paralysis, spinal affections, fever, diseased joints, surgical operations, consumptive and other invalids. The comfort of these mattresses is greater than can be well conceived. They are easily managed, being simply placed

on an ordinary bedstead. Orders by telegraph or otherwise immediately attended to—Hooper, sole maker, 7 Pall-mall east, 55 Grosvenor-street.

The claims made for the contemporary waterbed are just as extravagant, even though the ills it is said to alleviate are almost all different. The 1970s waterbed is said to be "ideal for overweight people . . . a must for long-term convalescents, cardiac and stroke patients . . . perfect for pregnant women . . . an absolute necessity for poor circulation." The manufacturers have no compunction about knocking the opposition: "A conventional bed may harbour millions of germs. A waterbed is *naturally hygienic.* A conventional bed actually *creates pressure* points, which cuts off blood flow and *causes* tossing and turning." So that's why I was tossing and turning!

A waterbed will support a ton of weight, proof of which is provided by a remarkable photograph of a morose and scabrous elephant sitting on one of these modern marvels looking as though he just couldn't wait for the photographer to go away so that he could return to his straw paillasse, for all its pressure points. I know that waterbeds don't leak, but irreverently, I was reminded of an infantile riddle:

Q. Why is an elephant sitting on an orange outside a synagogue?
A. He's waiting for the Jews to come out.

Before leaving waterbeds, I cannot resist telling you—in the words of the brochure—what it will do to your sex life:

Are these stories about waterbeds being so marvellous for sex, I mean are they really . . . I mean does it really sort of help out and . . . I mean . . .
Yes.

It has to be admitted that even a short exposure to the sales blarney of bed manufacturers leaves one crying "a plague on all your beds." Yet the bed must rank as one of the most important of all purchases. Strangely, one bed manufacturer told me that his customers chose their beds far more on the color and pattern of the mattress ticking, which they will not see again from one year to another, than on the actual comfort and quality of the springs.

Beds do matter. We each of us have our own personal preferences. I disagree violently with Marie Stopes about the rubber mattress, which I consider to be the most important advance in the whole history of the bed. But I agree with her on another count. Like the princess and the pea, I find it impossible to sleep with a rubber undersheet. Once again, everything depends on the rest—disturbed or peaceful—of the sleeper.

Living with Insomnia

BY BERNARD LEVIN

When The Times *of London, partly to assist the compiling of this book, invited readers to contribute their insomniac tips, the correspondence columns were filled for weeks with helpful advice. It was left to Bernard Levin,* The Times' *star columnist, to bring the correspondence to a close with his own unique combination of provocation and irresistible common sense.*

Is Bernard Levin really an insomniac? He claims to be, though I have a suspicion that he may just be masquerading as one, and is in fact one of nature's regular short sleepers. If worry about sleep is the criterion, he certainly disqualifies himself. This does not, however, discredit the value of his advice. I wish that he cared a bit more for bedside books, but I am quite sure that the recommendation to use one's waking hours of the night is the single most constructive thought to be found in this section of the book. Bernard Levin, incidentally, is a bachelor. Those insomniacs who share a double bed will know why it's not always prudent to switch on the light and start to chew an apple . . .

~~~~~~~~~~~~~~~~~~~~~~~~~~~~~~~~~~~

That multi-headed polymath, the readers of *The Times* of London, recently appealed to for specifics against insomnia, have come up with a variety of proven remedies ranging from reading their own sermons to wrapping a pair of their Auntie Nellie's red flannel drawers round their necks before retiring (or did I imagine that one?). Amid the suggestions, however, some of which I strongly suspect were not seriously offered, was this comment from the Reverend R. Q. Nelson:

> I used to tell them [sufferers from insomnia] to go to bed neither very early nor very late and to be sure that they were warm and comfortable. Then came the crux. I also told them that in these circumstances it did not matter whether they slept or not. If I convinced them of this, I succeeded in curing them. If not, I failed.

I now have to sum up the debate by telling you that the cloth has got it right, and everybody else has got it wrong. If you think I speak a shade dogmatically, I present my credentials: I have been an insomniac all my adult life, and indeed with three exceptions—once when I was in hospital, drugged, following an operation, once after I had not been in a bed, let alone asleep, for two consecutive nights, and once in France on the first night of a desperately needed holiday —I have not, for the best part of a quarter of a century, *ever* had more than roughly two hours' unbroken sleep.

Mind, I do not say that I sleep only two hours a night, only that I do not sleep more than that length of time without waking up, and most of the stretches of sleep, on most nights, are considerably shorter. In any normal night, I will wake up anything from four or five times to a dozen or more. I have done this, as I say, for as long as I can remember (I have occasionally thought of starting life anew as a professional insomniac, and only the fact that I cannot believe that there are any openings in such a trade has prevented me), and experience has taught me that all remedies, from reciting the speeches of Mr. Wedgwood Benn to reciting the speeches of Mr. Wedgwood Benn backwards, are a waste of time. The truth of the matter is what the man of God hints at in his letter: there is no such thing as insomnia.

I am aware that such a statement will cause scepticism verging upon ribaldry, but I am right, for all that. The mind and the body will take—will insist on taking—as much sleep as they need for any individual and what causes the effects ascribed to insomnia, effects which can range from permanent tiredness to serious breakdown, is not the inability to sleep, but the inability to realize that it doesn't matter.

But it doesn't. All quantities of sleep prescribed as "normal" (there is even an old saying that goes "seven hours' sleep for a man, eight for a woman and nine for a fool") are nothing but old wives' tales; no two people have exactly the same metabolism, and it is on the individual's make-up that the amount of sleep he or she needs depends, not on any arbitrary, or supposedly scientific, length of time said to be proper for everybody.

But if it is true that no man, by taking thought, can add one cubit to his stature, it is equally true that no man, by saying that there is no such thing as insomnia, can add five minutes to the length of time he stays asleep o'nights. The problem is: how does a man make himself believe that it does not matter if he lies awake? Now comes the part to which you must pay especially close attention, for the soothsayer, in the memorable words of Mr. Frankie Howerd, is about to say the sooth. Not only are all the sheep-counting formulas wrong; those who seek sleep in them are looking in a direction exactly opposite to that in which the solution may be found. All such remedies are designed to *waste* the sleepless hours; the solution is, on the contrary, to *use* them. From emptiness comes panic, which is what causes the after-effects attributed to insomnia; but from fullness comes peace of mind, and—at the proper moment—sleep.

I always have several books beside my bed, and they are never anthologies or other "bedside books," but books I seriously want to read, and to read right through. If they constitute work (such as a book I am reviewing) so much the better; if notes have to be made, better still. When I wake up, unless I feel sufficiently drowsy to be sure of getting off again quickly, I switch the light on and read or work. The mind thus engaged, it ceases to worry about the fact that it is awake, and when it wishes to go to sleep again, it makes its wishes clear. By employing the "dead time" in a pointless or trivial fashion, the waker is certain to find worry slipping in between sheep, so to speak, and then farewell the tranquil mind, farewell content.

Comfort, in all this, is essential. Have a jug of water, or a stronger tipple if you feel like it, alongside; I always have an apple to chew (I remember trying to demand a dish of apples from the Englishless concierge in a Finnish hotel, entirely by sign-language, and failing hilariously—God knows what he thought I was asking for), since there is nothing less conducive to comfort than a mouth like the proverbial parrot's cage, and getting up to clean my teeth every time I awake would be going a lot too far.

I do not lay down my prescriptions to be followed to the letter; every sleepless reader can work out his or her own variations on my theme. But the important thing, as I say, is to stop worrying about being awake, and it is along the lines I have laid out that the solution to this artificial problem of worry will be found. By following my advice, you will either go to sleep or stop feeling terrible when you cannot. Thank you and goodnight.

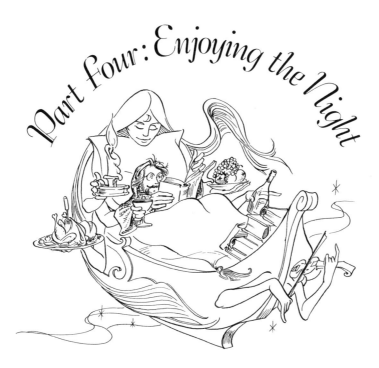

Part Four: Enjoying the Night

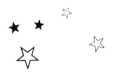

Making Light of Insomnia

Insomnia, like sex, sometimes needs to be taken seriously, but is always in danger of being taken too seriously. There's a sense in which the pursuit of the perfect night's rest is like the obsessional pursuit (with its attendant anxiety) to achieve the perfect simultaneous orgasm every time. How refreshing, and how necessary, are those who, like W. S. Gilbert and Ogden Nash (not to mention James Thurber, et al.) can look insomnia in the face—and laugh.

~~~~~~~~~~~~~~~~~~~~~~~~~~~

THE LORD CHANCELLOR'S SONG
by W. S. Gilbert

When you're lying awake with a dismal headache, and repose is taboo'd by anxiety, I conceive you may use any language you choose to indulge in, without impropriety;

For your brain is on fire—the bedclothes conspire of usual slumber to plunder you:

First your counterpane goes, and uncovers your toes, and your sheet slips demurely from under you;

Then the blanketing tickles—you feel like mixed pickles—so terribly sharp is the pricking,

And you're hot, and you're cross, and you tumble and toss till there's nothing 'twixt you and the ticking.

Then the bedclothes all creep to the ground in a heap, and you pick 'em all up in a tangle;

Next your pillow resigns and politely declines to remain at its usual angle!

Well, you get some repose in the form of a doze, with hot eye-balls and head ever aching,

But your slumbering teems with such horrible dreams that you'd very much better be waking;

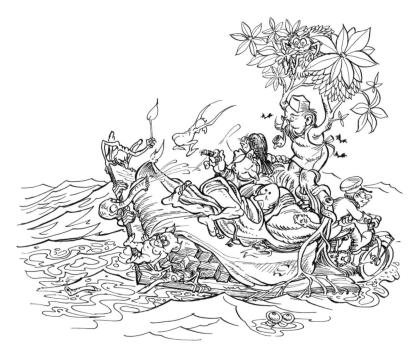

For you dream you are crossing the Channel, and tossing about in a steamer from Harwich—

Which is something between a large bathing machine and a very small second-class carriage—

And you're giving a treat (penny ice and cold meat) to a party of friends and relations—

They're a ravenous horde—and they all came on board at Sloane Square and South Kensington Stations.

And bound on that journey you find your attorney (who started that morning from Devon);

He's a bit undersized, and you don't feel surprised when he tells you he's only eleven.

Well, you're driving like mad with this singular lad (by the by, the ship's now a four-wheeler),

And you're playing round games, and he calls you bad names when you tell him that "ties pay the dealer"

But this you can't stand, so you throw up your hand, and you find you're as cold as an icicle,

In your shirt and your socks (the black silk with gold clocks), crossing Salisbury Plain on a bicycle:

And he and the crew are on bicycles too—which they've somehow or other invested in—

And he's telling the tars all the particu*lars* of a company he's interested in—

It's a scheme of devices, to get at low prices all goods from cough mixtures to cables

(Which tickled the sailors), by treating retailers as though they were all vege*ta*bles—

You get a good spadesman to plant a small tradesman (first take off his boots with a boot-tree),

And his legs will take root, and his fingers will shoot, and they'll blossom and bud like a fruit-tree—

From the greengrocer tree you get grapes and green pea, cauliflower, pineapple, and cranberries,

While the pastrycook plant cherry brandy will grant, apple puffs, and three-corners, and Banburys—

The shares are a penny, and ever so many are taken by Rothschild and Baring,

And just a few are allotted to you, you awake with a shudder despairing—

You're a regular wreck, with a crick in your neck, and no wonder you snore, for your
head's on the floor, and you've needles and pins from your soles to your shins, and
your flesh is a-creep, for your left leg's asleep, and you've cramp in your toes, and
a fly on your nose, and some fluff in your lung, and a feverish tongue, and a thirst
that's intense, and a general sense that you haven't been sleeping in clover;
But the darkness has passed, and it's daylight at last, and the night has been long—
ditto ditto my song—and thank goodness they're both of them over!

(From *Iolanthe*)

THE STILLY NIGHT: A SOPORIFIC REFLECTION
by Ogden Nash

He unwinds himself from the bedclothes each morn and piteously proclaims that he
didn't sleep a wink, and she gives him a glance savage and murderous
And replies that it was she who didn't close an eye until cockcrow because of his swinish
slumber as evidenced by his snores continuous and stertorous,
And his indignation is unconcealed,
He says she must have dreamed that one up during her night-long sweet repose, which
he was fully conscious of because for eight solid hours he had listened to her
breathing not quite so gentle as a zephyr on a flowery field.
The fact is that she did awaken twice for brief intervals and he was indeed asleep and
snoring, and he did awaken similarly and she was indeed unconscious and breathing miscellaneously,
But they were never both awake simultaneously.
Oh, sleep it is a blessed thing, but not to those wakeful ones who watch their mates
luxuriating in it when they feel that their own is sorely in arrears.
I am certain that the first words of the Sleeping Beauty to her prince were, "You *would*
have to kiss me just when I had dropped off after tossing and turning for a hundred
years."

Brain Games

Mental exercises certainly distract the mind, but do they actually assist sleep? One insomniac told me that she took pains to avoid them because they kept her mind active. I asked her what tracks her mind ran on otherwise, and she admitted that her most common habit was to contemplate gloomily all the lost opportunities of her life. She wasn't of course alone in this: many of us, lonely, unhappy or in stress, find ourselves following well-trodden and muddy paths of accusation or self-accusation. I'm inclined to think that any activity is preferable to that. The chief virtue of brain games is that they keep the mind occupied in a psychologically harmless way. If sleep seems to be held at bay, it may be because the individual doesn't need all that much sleep anyway. Personally, as a regular 4 a.m. player of the kind of games described below, I find that a session of compiling crossword clues, for instance, makes me much less of a tosser and turner than worrying about work, and sooner or later, my mind has had enough of its early-morning exercise, and I drop off once again.

By far the most popular of the ways of exercising the mind suggested by correspondents were alphabetical games of one kind or another. Making lists under each letter of the alphabet in turn was the most common of all, and the subjects for such lists are plainly inexhaustible: places you have visited, villages or towns in your neighborhood or in a particular state or county, rivers, animals, birds, vegetables, fruit, trees, flowers, colors, plays, films, famous artists or writers, occupations, boys' names, girls' names, names of kings or presidents. And there are of course plenty of other kinds of lists you can concoct if you are a list maker: the number of operas you have heard, the number of airports you have visited, the number of boys' names ending with -bert or girls' names ending with -lyn. Or you can count the number of a's and b's and c's in the Lord's Prayer ("I don't think God would mind," wrote the author of this idea). And so on, ad infinitum.

Here are some other alphabetical games to play if you are not a list maker. You can compose sentences with the same initial letter to each word, or telegrams with each word starting with successive letters of the alphabet. You can think of famous people with the initials AA, followed by AB, AC, etc., or alternatively, by BB, CC, etc. Or you can choose a general topic, such as Airport or Hospital, and then go through the alphabet to find suitable word associations: Airplane, Baggage, Cargo, Departure, or Ambulance, Bed, Casualty, Drug. And I liked the idea of counting your blessings, starting with an A blessing, then a B blessing, until you attain the ultimate blessing of Z for Zeal.

If you tire of the alphabet, there is a plethora of verbal games to wile away the hours. You can make up crossword-puzzle clues, or think up particularly teasing anagrams. (Can you find another six-letter word from the letters of c-h-e-s-t-y* or a ten-letter word from r-o-a-s-t m-u-l-e-s? †) You can see how many

*Scythe.
†Somersault.

160

words of three letters or more you can make from any five- or six-letter word. Or how many three-letter words end in y. Or which combination of four letters gives you the most four-letter words.* Or how many combinations of consonants you can find in which, by substituting each of the vowels in turn, you can make complete words—as in bag, beg, big, bog, bug. A final solution, one correspondent suggested, was to spell Czechoslovakia backward.

The world of mathematics offers another field of limitless diversion. If you are not good at spelling backward, you can always count backward. Someone told me his favorite sleep remedy was to count down from five hundred in threes and that he had never yet reached zero. He should be so lucky . . . You can pick a three-figure number at random and find out whether it's prime. You can set yourself all manner of multiplication and division problems. Or if you like counting money, you can work out the difference between the interest on a given sum when compounded quarterly at 4 1/2 percent for five years and simple interest at 5 percent for five years. If all else fails, you can always work out your tax returns in your head . . .

~~~~~~~~~~~~~~~~~~~~~~~~~~~~~

The following essay by Thurber is for those addicted to spending their night hours roaming across the limitless prairie of the alphabet. Readers who haven't the taste for these intriguing but pointless mental exercises had better skip this piece and the one that follows.

~~~~~~

*Post, stop, pots, opts, spot, tops.

THE WATCHERS OF THE NIGHT
by James Thurber

Most of the people I like, or love, or can barely stand are between the ages of forty-five and sixty-five, give or take a year or two at either end, and only about three of them are capable any longer of achieving what was once casually called, and is now wistfully called, a good night's rest. For ours is the age of the four A's: anxiety, apprehension, agonizing, and aspirin. People are smoking more and enjoying it less, drinking more and feeling it more, and waking around three in the morning to lie there gloomily staring at the mushroom-shaped ceiling, listening for the approaching drone of enemy bombers, and thinking of death but dressing it in the raiment of lyric or metaphor: the gate in the garden wall, the putting out to sea, the mother of beauty, the fog in the throat, the ruffian on the stair, the man in the white coat, the sleep that rounds our little lives.

If a husband wakes at three o'clock in the morning—once fondly known as the hour of a melody that Scott Fitzgerald called sweetly sad—he is not going to be able to lie there agonizing alone, the way his wife can, and frequently does. If they are in New York, which has an average of twelve dozen fire alarms every twenty-four hours, the wakeful husband will hear, sooner or later, the screaming of fire-engine sirens, which do not sound like heroic robots courageously rushing to a scene of disaster but like panicky monsters fleeing from this our life, shrieking hysterically in abject fear. It is at this moment in the dead of night that Papa usually feigns a nightmare in order to wake Mama and enjoy her warm scorn and her comforting scolding for interrupting her sleep. He will now be able to drop off again in a few minutes, but she will lie there, stark-staring awake, long enough to finish one or two mystery novels or to write, in her head, anywhere from five to fifteen letters of objection, correction, criticism, rebuttal, or denial, none of which she ever actually gets down on paper. All this has led to the sale and use of something like sixty-five million tranquillizing pills every year in this jumpy nation of ours.

I have joined the fifteen million people in the United States who are sixty-five years old or older, and for a good, or bad, five years I have been a three o'clock waker. I dread, as much as anyone else, the white watches of the woeful night, but, unlike most of my insomniac friends and enemies, I often think of the thousands of others who are also lying awake, and during the day I sometimes ask a few of them what they think about when they can't get back to sleep. One man, an architect and artist, says he starts with the town of Azusa, California, and moves eastward, a town and a letter of the alphabet at a time, hoping to doze off before he reaches Zanesville, Ohio. Another man, an overworked literary agent, makes up imaginary baseball teams, and is just now nocturnally engaged in forming one out of players whose names are the same as the names of occupations —Baker, Chandler, Tinker, and the like. No woman, of course, allows herself to fall into such a strange system of seeking sleep, for she is wise enough to know that a practice of that kind is a stimulant and not a soporific.

Since I have no mental discipline to speak of when I am horizontal, and little enough when I am upright, my conscious mind leads me into all kinds of sleep-murdering snarls. The other night, for example, I began with "We supply watchmen to watch men you want watched," and slowly built it up like this: "We supply watchwatchmen to watch watchmen watching men you want watched. We supply watchwomen to watch watchwatchmen watching watchmen watching men you want watched. We supply wristwatches for witchwatchers watching witches Washington wishes watched." At this point I woke Mama, and was asleep again by three forty-five, while she was awake long enough to reread *Trent's Last Case* and *The Murder of Roger Ackroyd.* For years now, I have kept myself awake while courting unconsciousness by tinkering with words and letters of the alphabet and spelling words backward. I am not going to spell anything backward in this piece except "pingpong" and one other expression we shall come to later. "Ping-pong," a trade name for table tennis, was presumably selected for its supposed onomatopoeic effect, but I submit that "gnip-gnop" is much more successful, that it really sounds like a game in progress. Another system of mine, which truly straight-arms sleep, is to rewrite, or paraphrase, Poe's *The Raven* from the viewpoint of the bird instead of that of the man.

> Once upon a daybreak dreary,
> While I fluttered sleek and cheery,
> Over many a granule of ungarnered corn,
> Suddenly there came a moaning, as of someone loudly groaning,
> Groaning at the thought of morn.

This version ends up with the raven trapped on the pallid bust of Pallas just above the chamber door. In other words, the unfortunate bird, lured into the sleepless scholar's chamber, has become a room raven. It was but the mental work of half an hour to figure—nay, to prove—that the raven speaks English with a foreign accent, and you can find this out for yourself simply by spelling "room raven" backward, beginning with the second word. This, to be sure, gets neither me nor you (nor Poe and the raven) anywhere except into the bad habit of mental left-reading in bed at night, and I guess I'm sorry I brought it up. (If Poe had rewritten *The Raven* in order to retract something, the result would have been a palinode, I thought you might want to know.)

For those watchers of the night who wake at the old Scott Fitzgerald hour and know darn well they are not going to get to sleep again, I suggest a ramble, a fascinating safari, through one of the letters of the alphabet. I have for weeks now been exploring the sixteenth letter of the alphabet, and have had more fun than a barrel of money (a barrel of monkeys is never fun but often, I should imagine, sheer hell, especially for the monkeys at the bottom of the barrel).

The letter "P," that broad, provocative expanse between "O" and "Q," is one of the most ambivalent of all the twenty-six, for in it one finds pleasure and pain, peace and pandemonium, prosperity and poverty, power and pusillanimity, plethora and paucity, pornography and prudery, purity and prurience, public and private, pastime and punishment, the patrician and the proletarian, and on and on, words without end.

Wanderers in the wide verbal terrain between "O" and "Q," with its panorama of plain and prairie, plateau and palisade, peninsula and promontory, can get on their horses and ride off in any one of all directions. It is well known, thanks to Clarence Day, that it is the wife, it is the home, that will not let the sailor roam and keeps the pioneer in town. This being the case, the wakeful captive husband is likely to see how far he can get from home and Mama, in fancy and fantasy. I play a night game called place-to-place, or around-the-world-in-eighty-names. The goal, a hopeless one, is to recall fourscore place names that strike no alarm bells in the memory. I hear none in Punxsutawney, or Papeete, or Irvin Cobb's Paducah, but from there on man and nature have made the going tough with Pakistan, Peiping, Panama, Pompeii, and there are still seventy-two more to come. It isn't easy to think only of Picardy's shining roses, or of the poppies of Provence, for both places are stained with blood as well as blossoms. The nocturnal wanderer, if he really wants to get his mind off himself and his era, might combine places and pastimes, and linger peacefully, for a little while, anyway, playing parcheesi in Put-in-Bay, post office in Perth Amboy, pinochle in Point Pleasant, polo in Paraguay, poker near Popocatepetl, pedro in Peru, and pigs-in-clover in Port Chester, but the chances of dozing off while wrestling with these imaginary dualities are slim. You are likely to get in deeper and deeper, until you are playing pillow with a pretty poetess in Patchen Place, or pitching pennies with the Pittsburgh Pirates in a pitter-patter of rain outside the Pitti Palace. (Select your own town for prisoner's base, pussy-wants-a-corner, and philopena—a playful practice, also known as "forfeits," which the Germans call *Vielliebchen,* or sweetheart.)

There are some wonderfully pixillated people in Bulfinch and in the *Oxford Classical Dictionary:* Pandora, the bungling busy-fingers who let all hell out of her hope chest; Proteus, the quick-change artist, who had more semblances than Ed Wynn had hats; and Phaethon, patron saint of the hot-rodsters of today, who drove the chariot of the sun wildly through the skies. Then there was my special pet, Phryne, a courtesan who lived in the fourth century B.C. Once, "she laid aside her garments, let down her hair, and stepped into the sea in the sight of the people." On another occasion, she was brought to trial on a charge of having profaned the Eleusinian mysteries. Things looked pretty bad for her until her counsel "rent her robe and displayed her bosom, which so moved her judges that they acquitted her." Our sixteenth letter played a prominent part in her life—a statue of her was made by Praxiteles, her story was told by Pliny, and it was during the festival of Poseidon that she stepped naked into the sea.

The marvellous sixteenth letter of the alphabet is, to be sure, the country of predicament, plight, problem, perplexity, pickle, pretty pass, puzzle, pit, pitfall, and palindrome. There are many night-time palindromists in America, caught, or hooked, by the lure of searching for words or phrases that are spelled the same way forward and backward. Among the oldest are "Madam I'm Adam," and "lewd did I live, & evil I did dwel," which are child's play compared to such a new beauty as "a man, a plan, a canal, Panama." I am in touch with several palindrome addicts who have come up with things like "deified," "he goddam mad dog, eh?," and a few longer flights in which slight misspellings are permissible, one of them being the ten-word boast of a queen who drank beer after rum and still managed a good night's rest: "Piel's lager on red rum did murder no regal sleep."

There is one pre-eminent category of "P" that lifts the heart, inspires the spirit, and fortifies faith in man, even if you don't get back to sleep, and that is the category of the pioneers, the pilgrims, and the pathfinders, the immortal heroes of the Shining Quests: Sir Percivale and the Holy Grail; Sir Palamedes and the Questing Beast; Perseus and the dread Medusa; Peary and the North Pole; Ponce and the Fountain of Youth; Marco Polo and the trade routes to the East; Pickett, who tried to reach Washington through the center of Meade's line; Pollux, who helped find the Golden Fleece; Porthos, one of the picaresque posse that set out in pursuit of the Queen's diamonds; the brothers Piccard, who hunted for everything, in ballocas and bathyspheres; and I almost forgot Plato, who searched for truth (Pontius Pilate just asked what it was, and doesn't belong here), and Pythagoras, who sought to trace the flight of the human soul.

The nocturnal wanderer in the prolific consonant should avoid the area of disease, both physical and mental, if he doesn't want to scare himself to death. "P" seems to be afflicted with almost all of the major ailments and maladies of mind and body, so it's fortunate that it also has the physician, psychologist, psychiatrist, pharmacist, pathologist and literally dozens of their colleagues, as well as the pope, preacher, parson, priest, prelate, primate, padre, and a helpful host of others.

Let us glance at some of the reasons for the presence of these people, at the risk of becoming a touch scholarly but, I hope, not stuffy. In the Old English or Anglo-Saxon vocabulary, the fewest words began with "P." It had only half as many as the letter "I" and even fewer than "Y." Then, as man prattled on, the letter became the third largest in the alphabet, with only "S" and "C" exceeding it in output. The triad formed by these three letters gives our vocabulary one-third of all its words. The accessions were Germanic and Teutonic, to begin with, and then it began receiving the rich heritage of French and the other Romance languages, and Greek and Latin, especially words beginning with Latin prefixes. There were other additions, too, as time went on, from what the indispensable *Oxford English Dictionary* calls "the Oriental, African, American, and other remote languages." Furthermore, many additions of words beginning with "P" are of unknown origin, which causes the *O.E.D.* to observe: "P thus presents probably a greater number of unsolved etymological problems than any other letter."

I suggest that a married couple, in one bed or twin beds, sedulously avoid playing the letter game together in the middle of the night. Mama is sure to get sore because her spouse has ignored Lily Pons, Mary Pickford, Patti Page,

Portia, Mrs. Pankhurst, Mrs. Potter Palmer, Pocahontas, Molly Pitcher, and all the other great ladies of the letter, and she is more than likely to defend Pandora as not being a pixie at all, but a lady more important than Prometheus, who started a lot of trouble by bringing fire to our poor planet. Papa will claim that Pandora was a mischievous cutup, comparable to the poltergeist, and far less interesting than the porpoise, that chuckling prankster of the sea, or the penguin, the playbird of the polar parts. The argument, as you can perceive, is capable of going on until cockcrow.

Prisoners of parody and paraphrase, prostrate and pillowed, are prone to tinker with the world and words of Lewis Carroll at the slightest prod or provocation. And so, my very latest nights have been plagued by persistent poppcockalorum like this: "Twas throllog and the siren tones did shriek and gibber in the night, all menace were the bomberdrones, and the mom wrath outright." But enough of this, and if you should ever be able to fall asleep at night from now on, pleasant dreams.

AINMOSNI
by Roger Angell

There are many alternative tracks available to those who enjoy what Thurber calls "an alphabetical safari." The anagram trail is well frequented, but the path of the palindrome, celebrated here by the New Yorker *writer Roger Angell, also offers endless opportunities for the midnight word hunter.*

~~~~~~~~~~~~~~~~~~~~~~~~~~~~~~~~~~~~~

Insomnia is my baby. We have been going steady for a good twenty years now, and there is no hint that the dull baggage is ready to break off the affair. Three or four times a week, somewhere between three and six in the morning, this faulty thermostat inside my head clicks to "On," raising my eyelids with an almost audible clang and releasing a fetid blast of night thoughts. Sighing, I resume my long study of the bedroom ceiling and the uninteresting shape (a penguin? an overshoe?) that the street light, slanting through the window, casts on the closet door, while I review various tedious strategems for recapturing sleep. If I am resolute, I will arise and robe myself, stumble out of the bedroom (my wife sleeps like a Series E government bond), turn on the living-room lights, and take down a volume from my little shelf of classical pharmacopeia. George Eliot, James, and Montaigne are Nembutals, slow-acting but surefire. Thoreau, a dangerous Seconal-Demerol bomb, is reserved for emergencies; thirty minutes in the Walden beanfield sends me back to bed at a half run, fighting unconsciousness all the way down the hall. Too often, however, I stay in bed, under the delusion that sleep is only a minute or two away.

This used to be the time for Night Games, which once worked for me. I would invent a No-Star baseball game, painstakingly selecting two nines made up of the least exciting ballplayers I could remember (mostly benchwarmers with the old Phillies and Senators) and playing them against each other in the deserted stadium of my mind. Three or four innings of walks, popups, foul balls, and messed-up double plays, with long pauses for rhubarbs and the introduction of relief pitchers, would bring on catalepsy. Other nights, I would begin a solo round of golf (I am a terrible golfer) on some recalled course. After a couple of pars and a brilliantly holed birdie putt, honesty required me to begin playing my real game, and a long search for my last golf ball, horribly hooked into the cattails to the left of the sixth green, would uncover, instead, a lovely Spalding Drowz-Rite. In time, however, some perverse sporting instinct began to infect me, and my Night Games became hopelessly interesting. As dawn brightened the bedroom, a pinch-hitter would bash a line drive that hit the pitcher's rubber and rebounded crazily into a pail of water in the enemy dugout, scoring three runs and retying the game, 17–17, in the twenty-first inning; my drive off the fourteenth tee, slicing toward a patch of tamaracks, would be seized in midair by an osprey and miraculously dropped on the green, where I would begin lining up my putt just as the alarm went off. I had to close up the ballpark and throw away my clubs; I was bushed.

It was an English friend of mine, a pink-cheeked poet clearly accustomed to knocking off ten hours' sleep every night, who got me into real small-hours trouble. He observed me yawning over a lunchtime Martini one day and drew forth an account of my ridiculous affliction. "I can help you, old boy," he announced. "Try palindromes."

"Palindromes?" I repeated.

"You know—backward-forward writing," he went on. "Reads the same both ways. You remember the famous ones: 'Madam, I'm Adam.' 'Able was I ere I saw Elba.' 'A man, a plan, a canal: Panama.' The Elba one is supposed to be about Napoleon. Here—I'll write it for you. You see, 'Able' backward is 'Elba,' and—"

"I know, I know," I snapped. "But what's that got to do with not sleeping? Am I supposed to repeat them over and over, or what?"

"No, that's no good. You must make up your own. Nothing to it. Begin with two-way words, and soon you'll be up to sentences. I do it whenever I can't sleep —'sleep' is 'peels,' of course—and in ten minutes I pop right off again. Never fails. Just now, I'm working on a lovely one about Eliot, the poet. 'T. Eliot, top bard . . .' it begins, and it ends, 'drab pot toilet.' Needs a bit of work in the middle, but I'll get it done one of these nights."

I was dubious, but that night, shortly after four, I began with the words. In a few minutes, I found "gulp plug" (something to do with bass fishing) and "live evil," and sailed off into the best sleep I had enjoyed in several weeks. The next night brought "straw warts" and "repaid diaper," and, in time, a long if faintly troubled snooze ("ezoons"). I was delighted. My palindromic skills improved rapidly, and soon I was no longer content with mere words. I failed to notice at first that, like all sedatives, this one had begun to weaken with protracted use; I was doubling and tripling the dose, and my intervals given over to two-way cogitation were stretching to an hour or more. One morning, after a mere twenty minutes of second shut-eye, I met my wife at the breakfast table and announced, " 'Editor rubs ward, draws burro tide.' "

"Terrific," she said unenthusiastically. "I don't get it. I mean, what does it *mean?*"

"Well, you see," I began, "there's this editor in Mexico who goes camping with his niece, and—"

"Listen," she said. "I think you should take a phenobarb tonight. You look terrible."

It was about six weeks later when, at five-fifteen one morning, i discovered the Japanese hiding in my pajamas. "Am a Jap," he said, bowing politely, and then added in a whisper, "Pajama." I slept no more. Two nights later, at precisely four-eleven, when "Repins pajama" suddenly yielded "Am a Jap sniper," I sprang out of bed, brewed myself a pot of strong coffee, and set to work with pencil and paper on what had begun to look like a war novel. A month later, trembling, hollow-eyed, and badly strung out on coffee and Dexamyl, I finished the epic. It turned out that the thing wasn't about a Japanese at all; it was a long telegram composed by a schizophrenic war veteran who had been wounded at Iwo Jima and was now incarcerated in some mental hospital. (This kind of surprise keeps happening when you are writing palindromes, a literary form in which the story line is controlled by the words rather than the author.) Experts have since told me that my barely intelligible pushmi-pullyu may be the longest palindrome in the English language:

MARGE, LET DAM DOGS IN. AM ON SATIRE: VOW I AM CAIN. AM ON SPOT, AM A JAP SNIPER. RED, RAW MURDER ON G.I.! IGNORE DRUM. (WARDER REPINS PAJAMA TOPS.) NO MANIAC, MA! IWO VERITAS: NO MAN IS GOD.   —MAD TELEGRAM

My recovery was a protracted one, requiring a lengthy vacation at the seashore, daily exercise, warm milk on retiring, and eventually a visit to the family psychiatrist. The head-candler listened to my story ("Rot-cod . . ." I began), then wrote out a prescription for a mild sedative (I murmured, "slip pils") and swore me to total palindromic abstinence. He told me to avoid Tums, Serutan, and men named Otto. "Only right thinking can save you," he said severely. "Or rather, *left-to-right* thinking."

I tried, I really tried. For more than a year, I followed the doctor's plan faithfully, instantly dropping my gaze whenever I began to see "POTS" and "KLAW" on traffic signs facing me across the street, and plugging away at my sleepy-time books when I was reafflicted with the Big Eye. I had begun to think that mine might be a total cure when, just two weeks ago, nodding over "Walden" again, I came upon this sentence: "We are conscious of an animal in us, which awakens in proportion as our higher nature slumbers. It is reptile and sensual, and perhaps cannot be wholly expelled . . ."

"Ah-ha!" I muttered, struck by the remarkable pertinence of this thought to my own nocturnal condition. Thoreau himself had said it; I could never quite escape. To prove the point, I repeated my exclamation, saying it backward this time.

I did not entirely give way to my reptile. Remembering my near-fatal bout with the telegram, I vowed to limit myself entirely to revising and amplifying existing palindromes—those famous chestnuts recited to me by my English friend. The very next night, during a 4 A.M. rainstorm, I put my mind to "A man, a plan, a canal: Panama." Replacing de Lesseps with a female M.I.T. graduate, I achieved "A *woman*, a plan, a canal: Panamowa," which was clearly inadequate; she sounded more like a ballerina. Within a few minutes, however, a dog trotted out of the underbrush of my mind—it was a Pekinese—and suddenly redesigned the entire isthmus project: "A dog, a plan, a canal: pagoda." I went to sleep.

Napoleon led me into deeper waters. Bedwise by night light, I envisioned him as a fellow-sufferer, a veteran palindromist who must have been transfixed with joy to find the island of his first exile so brilliantly responsive to his little perversion. But what if the allies had marooned him on a *different* island in

1814? Various possibilities suggested themselves: "A dum reb was I ere I saw Bermuda." . . . "No lava was I ere I saw Avalon." . . . "Lana C. LaDaug was I ere I saw Guadalcanal." None would do; the Emperor's aides, overhearing him, would conclude that the old boy had fallen victim to aphasia. A night or two later, I replaced Boney on Elba and retinued him with a useful and highly diversified staff of officers and loyal friends—a Rumanian, a female camp follower, a Levantine, and a German. These accompanied the Emperor by turns during his habitual evening walks along the cliffs, each feigning awe and delight as the impromptu musing of the day fell down from his lips. "Uncomfortable was I ere I saw Elba, Trofmocnu," he confessed to the first. To the female, smiling roguishly and chucking her under the chin, he murmured, "Amiable was I ere I saw Elba, Ima." The next evening, made gloomy by the rabbinical sidekick, he changed to "Vegetable was I ere I saw Elba, Tegev." He cheered up with the burly Prussian, declaiming: "Remarkable was I ere I saw Elba, Kramer!" but, finding the same man on duty the following night (the list had run out, and new duty rosters were up), he reversed himself, whining, "*Un*remarkable was I ere I saw Elba, Kramer, *nu?*"

That seemed to exhaust Elba (and me), and during the wee hours of last week I moved along inevitably to "Madam, I'm Adam." For some reason, this jingle began to infuriate me. (My new night journeys had made me irritable and suspicious; my wife seemed to be looking at me with the same anxious expression she had worn when I was fighting the Jap sniper, and one day I caught her trying to sneak a telephone call to the psychiatrist.) Adam's salutation struck me as being both rude and uninformative. At first, I attempted to make the speaker more civilized, but he resisted me: "Good day, Madam, I'm Adam Yaddoog." . . . "Howdy, Madam, I'm Adam Y. Dwoh." . . . "*Bonjour*, Madam, I'm Adam Roujnob." No dice. Who *was* this surly fellow? I determined to ferret out his last name, but the first famous Adam I thought of could only speak after clearing his throat ("*Htims*, Madam, I'm Adam Smith"), and the second had to introduce himself just after falling down a flight of stairs ("Yksnilomray!

. . . Madam, I'm Adam Yarmolinsky"). Then, at exactly six-seventeen yesterday morning, I cracked the case. I was so excited that I woke up my wife. She stared at me, blurry and incredulous, as I stalked about the bedroom describing the recent visit of a well-known congressman to Wales. He had gone there, I explained, on a fact-finding trip to study mining conditions in the ancient Welsh collieries, perhaps as necessary background to the mine-safety bills now

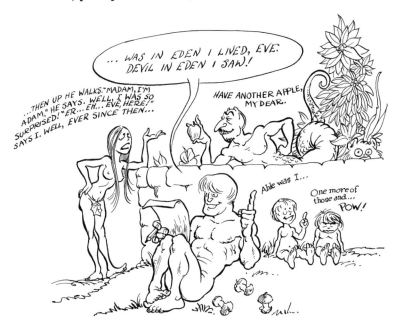

pending in Washington. Being a highly professional politician, he boned up on the local language during the transatlantic plane trip. The next morning, briefcase and homburg in hand, he tapped on the door of a miner's cottage in Ebbw Vale, and when it was opened by a lady looking very much like Sara Allgood in *How Green Was My Valley*, he smiled charmingly, bowed, and said, "*Llewopnotyalc*, Madam, I'm Adam Clayton Powell."

When I got home last night, I found a note from my wife saying that she had gone to stay with her mother for a while. Aware at last of my nearness to the brink, I called the psychiatrist, but his answering service told me that he was away on a month's vacation. I dined forlornly on hot milk and Librium and was asleep before ten . . . and awake before three. Alone in bed, trembling lightly, I restudied the penguin (or overshoe) on the wall, while my mind, still unleashed, sniffed over the old ashpiles of canals, islands, and Adams. Nothing there. Nothing, that is, until seven-twelve this morning, when the beast unearthed, just under the Panama Canal, the small but glittering prize, "Suez . . . Zeus!" I sat bolt upright, clapping my brow, and uttered a great roar of delight and despair. Here, I could see, was a beginning even more promising than the Jap sniper. Released simultaneously into the boiling politics of the Middle East and the endless affairs of Olympus, I stood, perhaps, at the doorway of the greatest palindromic adventure of all time—one that I almost surely would not survive. "No!" I whimpered, burying my throbbing head beneath the pillows. "No, no!" Half smothered in linen and sleeplessness, I heard my sirens reply. "On!" they called. "On, on!"

PILLOW PUZZLES

This section is for those who prefer to be set mental tasks rather than make them up for themselves. Charles Dodgson, mathematical lecturer at Christ Church, Oxford, but better known by his pen name, Lewis Carroll, was the first to publish a collection of mental conundrums specially designed for the comfort of insomniacs. In the Preface to Pillow Problems *he offers a classic defense of this sort of cerebral gym:*

> The word "comfort" may perhaps sound out of place in connection with so entirely *intellectual* an occupation; but it will, I think, come home to many who have known what it is to be haunted by some worrying subject of thought which no effect of will is able to banish. Again and again I have said to myself, on lying

down at night after a day embittered by some vexatious matter, "I will *not* think of it any more!" And in another ten minutes I have found myself once more in the very thick of this miserable business, and torturing myself to no purpose with all the old troubles.

Now it is not possible—this, I think, all psychologists will admit—by any effort of volition, to carry out the resolution, "I will *not* think of so-and-so." (Witness the common trick, played on a child, of saying "I'll give you a penny, if you'll stand in that corner for five minutes and *not once* think of strawberry jam." No human child ever yet won the tempting wager.) But it *is* possible—as I am most thankful to know—to carry out the resolution "I *will* think of so-and-so." Once fasten the attention upon a subject so chosen, and you will find that the worrying subject, which you desire to banish, is *practically* annulled. It may recur from time to time —just looking in at the door so to speak; but it will find itself so coldly received, and will get so little attention paid to it, that it will, after a while, cease to be any worry at all.

Perhaps I may venture for a moment to use a more serious tone, and to point out that there are mental troubles much worse than mere worry, for which an absorbing subject of thought may serve as a remedy. There are sceptical thoughts, which seem for the moment to uproot the firmest faith; there are blasphemous thoughts which dart unbidden into the most reverent souls; there are unholy thoughts, which torture with their hateful presence the fancy that would fain be pure. Against all these some real mental *work* is a most helpful ally.

Lewis Carroll's puzzles are mathematically too sophisticated for the average reader. I prefer Ivan Morris and Edward de Bono. Ivan Morris is not only a distinguished Japanese scholar, he is also an inveterate scavenger of brain games. His book Pillow Book Puzzles *grades puzzles on the Michelin principle: one star for Brief Diversions, two for Hard Nuts and three for Herculeans. I have chosen two each from the first two grades and one from the last. Edward de Bono, the evangelist of lateral thinking, is one of the great puzzle makers of our time, and I have added a further five of his problems to the vintage five culled by Morris.*

All ten puzzles have in common that they can be read with the light on and then teased out in the dark. (Solutions, and some comments by Edward de Bono on his puzzles, start on page 180.)

~~~~~~~~~~~~~~~~~~~~~~~~~~~~~~~~~~~~~

1.

The Wettened Wrist Watches
★

Roger and Mabel go for a swim, both forgetting to remove their wrist watches. The watches are damaged. Roger's starts gaining thirty seconds a day and Mabel's stops entirely. If both of them decide never to set or repair their watches, which of the two will tell the exact time more often, and how much more often?

(Based on Lewis Carroll)

2.

Pints
★

With nothing but a three-pint and a five-pint container, how can you measure one pint of liquid? (There is an indefinite supply of liquid.)

3.

The Unemployed Professors
★ ★

Three professors of philosophy are seeking employment in a certain university. The dean informs them as follows: "I shall draw a blue or a white dot on each of your foreheads. If you see a white dot on anyone's forehead, please raise your right hand. As soon as you know your own color, please lower your hand."

He puts white dots on all three professors, and of course they all raise their hands. Fairly soon one of them, Professor Sol ("Ipy") Hoph, lowers his hand and declares, "Obviously I must have a white dot."

"How do you know?" asks the dean.

Professor Hoph's explanation wins him the job. How does he explain that he must have a white dot? (There are no mirrors in the room.)

4.
The Condemned Prisoner
★ ★

Warden: I regret to inform you officially that you will be hanged during the course of this month, but you will never know in advance which day it is to be.

Condemned prisoner: Splendid! That means that I shall never be hanged.

Warden: Bother! So it does.

Was the prisoner's optimism justified? If so, why? And how should the warden have worded his statement?

5.
The Road to Heaven
★ ★ ★

Reaching a fork in the road where one way leads to Heaven and the other to Hell, you encounter three shadowy figures. One of them (Gandhi) always tells the truth, another (Goebbels) never tells the truth, and the third (De Gaulle) sometimes tells the truth. It is impossible to distinguish among the three figures.

You are allowed two questions of the type that can be answered "Yes" or "No" to find out which way leads to Heaven. Both questions may be addressed to the same shadow or the two questions may be addressed to two different shadows.

6.

Gold and Lead

Equal lengths of gold and lead are balanced on the pans of a scale. The scale is immersed completely in water. What happens?

7.

Mirror-Writing

Leonardo da Vinci used to write his notes in mirror-writing. Could you use a typewriter to write in this manner?

8.

Slantwise

A painter has a visual defect which makes all vertical lines appear to slant to the left. What will his paintings look like?

9.

A Three-Mile Walk

A brother, a sister and a dog set out for a walk (walking speeds: boy 4 m.p.h., girl 3 m.p.h., dog 10 m.p.h.). The girl cannot keep up with her rude brother, who gradually draws ahead. The more polite dog is uncertain with whom he ought to stay and so moves continually back and forth from one to the other. The walk is three miles long and the boy naturally arrives home before his sister. How many miles has the dog actually covered?

10.

Chocolate Block

A bar of chocolate is three blocks wide by eight blocks long. If you are not allowed to double up pieces, what is the minimum number of breaks you would have to make in order to separate each block?

SOLUTIONS

1. *The Wettened Wrist Watches*

It will take 2 × 60 × 12 half-days, i.e., 720 days, for Roger's watch to show the exact time again. During these days Mabel's watch will have shown the correct time twice every twenty-four hours, that is, 1,440 times. So her watch will have shown the exact time almost 1,500 times more often than Roger's.

2. *Pints*

Fill the three-pint container; empty it into the five-pint container; fill the three-pint container again; empty it into the five-pint container until the latter is full; now one pint will remain in the three-pint container.

3. *The Unemployed Professors*

Let us call the other two professors A and B. Professor Hoph reasons as follows: "Suppose my dot is blue. Then Professor A must instantly realize that he is white (else why would Professor B be raising his hand?). Since Professor A has not in fact lowered his hand, my supposition must be incorrect. I am therefore white."

The following solution is also possible: "Assuming that a professor of philosophy would allow himself to go through the tomfoolery involved, he might also take for granted that all candidates were being tested in the same way. Therefore, if the other two have white dots and he did not, they were being given another test. Therefore he has a white dot."

4. *The Condemned Prisoner*

The prisoner is entirely correct. According to the warden's formula, the execution cannot possibly take place on the last day of the month, for if the prisoner survives until the last day but one, he must know that only one day remains for the execution (namely, the last day) and the warden has promised that he will never know the date of execution in advance. Since the last day of the month is thus ruled out, the last day but one is also impossible, for if the prisoner lives through the last day but two, he must realize that the only day left for the execution (the last day having been eliminated as a possibility) is the last day but one, and again the warden has said that he will never know in advance. Since the last two days of the month are disqualified, the last day but two is also disqualified by the same reasoning. Working backward according to this logic, the prisoner realizes that all the days of the month are ruled out.

Obviously the warden should have added the following words to his original statement: " . . . unless, of course, it is the last day." The prospect of being hanged, as Dr. Johnson remarked, concentrates the mind wonderfully.

5. *The Road to Heaven*

The real difficulty arises from the presence of someone who occasionally tells the truth, and the aim of the first question must be to "eliminate" him so that the second question can be directed to a shadow that is known to be consistently honest or dishonest.

First question: Let us call the three shadows A, B and C. This question is directed to A: "Is B more likely to tell the truth than C?" If the answer is "Yes," then if A is Gandhi, B is De Gaulle and C is Goebbels; if A is Goebbels, B is De Gaulle and C is Gandhi; if A is De Gaulle, B is either Gandhi or Goebbels, and C is either Gandhi or Goebbels. It will immediately be seen that in none of these three cases is C De Gaulle. Similarly, if the answer to the first question is "No," then in none of the three cases can B be De Gaulle. The second question is therefore addressed to C or B, depending on whether the answer to the first question was "Yes" or "No" respectively. You do not know whom you are addressing, but you can be certain that it is not De Gaulle.

Second question: "Would the shadow whose truth/lying habits are the exact opposite to yours say that the left-hand road leads to Heaven?" If the answer is "Yes," we know that the right-hand road leads to Heaven. For if you were addressing Gandhi, he would reply that his "opposite," i.e., Goebbels, would say that the left-hand road leads to Heaven, whereas, in fact, it is the right-hand road that goes there; alternatively, if you were addressing Goebbels, he would reply that his "opposite," Gandhi, would say that the left-hand road leads to Heaven, whereas he knows very well that what Gandhi would actually reply is that it is the right-hand road. In other words, the answer is the same regardless of whom you are questioning. Similarly, if the reply is "No," it means that the left-hand road leads to Heaven. (An alternative second question depends on the use of a double negative, as in "If you were asked whether the left-hand road leads to Heaven, would you reply in the affirmative?" If the left-hand road does in fact lead to Heaven, both Gandhi and Goebbels will answer "Yes" to this question; if it doesn't, they will both answer "No.")

6. *Gold and Lead*

Gold is heavier than lead, so a piece of gold will be smaller than an equal amount of lead. On immersion of the scales in water the lead will displace more water than the gold and hence will lose more weight. The scales will tilt down on the gold side.

Comment: Many people are too suspicious and suspect a catch. They fasten onto the equal weights of gold and lead and declare that they must remain balanced whatever happens. Under water, however, it is density that counts.

7. *Mirror-Writing*

Disconnect the ribbon and put into the typewriter a piece of paper backed by a piece of carbon paper with the inky side uppermost. The type keys will hit the paper on to the carbon and mirror-writing will appear on the underside of the paper.

Comment: One is so used to writing on the top of a piece of paper that many people never consider the possibility of writing on the underside. The problem is insoluble until one makes this jump.

8. *Slantwise*

The paintings would look perfectly normal. If the painter sees a telegraph pole as slanting, then in order for it to look right to him he would have to paint it vertically on his canvas.

Comment: One is not looking at the painter's view of the world but at the expression of that view which is just as external to the painter as the real world.

9. *A Three-Mile Walk*

If the walk is three miles long, then walking at 3 m.p.h., it must take the girl exactly one hour to finish it. Since the dog is moving while the girl is, the dog must be moving for one hour. At a speed of 10 m.p.h., the dog will have covered ten miles in one hour.

Comment: If you look at the problem in the obvious way and consider the distance moved by the dog it is very difficult. Looking at the problem in terms of time, not distance, makes it very easy.

10. *Chocolate Block*

Each break will produce one more piece than before the break. So to produce 24 separate pieces there will have to be 23 breaks.

Comment: By focusing attention on exactly what happens at each operation and deriving a principle, the problem is made very easy. Many people spend a long time trying to work it out mathematically.

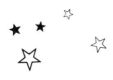

Nastier Nights Than Yours

All of us remember from our childhood that special delight which comes from being snug in a warm bed while a snowstorm or hurricane rages outside. It happens to be one of the rare pleasures that can be recaptured every time there's a gale blowing at bedtime. Even if the barometer is set fair, it is still possible to produce a similar glow from reading about perfectly awful nights that have been endured by the intrepid or the masochistic. Whether or not the accounts that follow—the gruesome adventures of a potholer and an Antarctic explorer—send the reader to sleep, they should help to make him grateful for the comfort of a warm bed with a roof overhead and a dry mattress beneath.

BEYOND TIME
by Michel Siffre

In 1962 Michel Siffre, a twenty-two-year-old French geologist, spent sixty-three days alone in a glaciated cave 375 feet beneath the surface of the earth in the Alpes Maritimes. His object was less speleological research than to explore the frontiers of man's physical and psychological endurance. Here is his account of life underground:

~~~~~~~~~~~~~~~~~~~~~~~~~~~~~~~~~~~~~

Until my survival experiment in the Scarasson Cavern no one had tried to survive for a protracted period in such a hostile environment: with a temperature constantly at or below freezing, an atmosphere saturated with humidity, shut off from sunlight (deemed indispensable to life), without any social or mechanical or cosmic points of reference to indicate the time of day or night, and all this endured in solitude.

During the two months I spent underground in the depths of the cavern, I kept a diary in which I noted down everything that happened during my physiological days—that is to say, between my periods of waking and sleeping. To begin with, I had hoped to write every evening a detailed account of what I had done. Soon, however, I found that by the time I was ready to go to sleep I could not at all remember what I had done, although the period of activity (my "day") had seemed very short. This loss of memory became so pronounced that it was sometimes hard for me to remember what I had done a few minutes before.

Time seemed to pass very quickly. As my diary shows, I thought it was August 20th when I was told that my experiment had lasted two months and that the date was actually September 17th. Time passed without my being aware of it in the darkness and silence. I felt I was on another planet; for the most part

I dwelt neither in the past nor in the future, but in the hostile present. In that environment everything was against me: the rocks that crashed down from time to time; the damp, chill atmosphere; the darkness. I waged a ceaseless combat with myself to surmount these terrors by sheer will power, and I owe my survival to that incessant battle.

From the minute I woke up, the torments began. In that glacial air it took courage to reach out of the more or less warm sleeping bag to turn on the light —an electric bulb of weak voltage clamped to the metal head of my camp bed. Usually I lay in the darkness for a while, gathering courage, hoping I might fall asleep again. Perhaps it was still the middle of the night: I had no way of knowing. Then, resolutely, I would reach out and press the button, shattering the dense darkness. My next duty took still more courage. According to our arrangements, I was to telephone the surface when I awoke, when I was ready to eat a meal, and when I was about to go to sleep; in this way my hazarded time of day could be checked against the actual time which those on guard must never tell me. I kept a chart of my subjective "time" and they kept a chart of the actual time. I have already stated this, but I repeat: throughout the time I spent in the Scarasson Cavern, I had no means whatsoever of knowing the day of the month or the hour of the day, and those on the surface were strictly forbidden to reveal them to me. My only way of estimating time was by means of my physiological functions, and these functions in man have been conditioned since the beginning of his existence on earth by the regular alternation of night and day, so we thought.

As it turned out, little by little a new biological rhythm was set up, similar to the rhythm to which astronauts of the future may be subjected in their long interplanetary voyages. Until this experiment of mine in 1962, experiments in voluntary isolation in conditions excluding variations of light and darkness had never exceeded one week. Perhaps it will be possible to extend the experiment beyond the two months that I held out without causing the crises of depression which have interrupted previous experiments.

The first words I pronounced on the telephone were the date and hour I presumed it to be and the amount of time I presumed had elapsed since my previous call. During the first days I had the impression that I slept a great deal —from twelve to thirteen hours; later on, I believed I was sleeping for shorter periods, six or seven hours.

As time went on, the telephone calls I had to put through upon waking up became a frightful ordeal. Rising was a harsh test of courage; the sleeping bag was the only place where I found relative comfort. By habit an early riser, I struggled against this torpor. I now believe that if I had given way to it I would not be alive to tell the story. Sometimes I lingered on in my warm nest and read a book. But reading in bed was not as luxurious as it sounds: one arm had to be outside the sleeping bag, and in a few minutes it became stiff with the cold. So then, I would partially dress. This took courage, as well. The outside of my sleeping bag was always damp, covered with fine water drops. At first I pulled on my woolen shirt that lay nearby, shuddering, for it, too, was damp and cold. Then I found I could warm it slightly before putting it on by dragging it into my sleeping bag with me. But it was too cold to touch with my warm body.

When finally I courageously dressed and got out of bed, I heated water in a basin, always the same one, which I never washed and which stood outside the entrance to the tent. While the water heated, I studied my time graph and tried to bring it "up to date"—after only a few days down below I was not sure what the date was. Intuitively I felt that my time recordings were wrong and certainly did not coincide with my physiological rhythms of hunger and sleepiness, but were often quite wide of the mark. Sometimes, for instance, I was subjectively convinced that it was the middle of the night; yet I felt hungry and in need of activity. Therefore, I argued with myself, it must be the middle of the day. Tortured with these scruples, I was uncertain how to mark my time graph.

Sometimes I awakened feeling in perfect form, physically and mentally; but at other times I woke up suffering so acutely from the cold and the loneliness that even talking to the men on the surface by telephone did not seem to cheer me, although I forced myself not to betray my melancholy mood to them. (They now tell me that, despite my efforts to sound cheerful, they always sensed my depressed moods.) I will confess that my periods of depression were often brought on by some particularly fearful cave-in of rocks and ice. Or perhaps by a near-accident, as, for instance, exploring the lower end of the glacier, I very nearly slipped and crashed into the void. What a death that would have been! Either I would have died of the cold or, transfixed on a jagged rock, would have suffered a slow agony. On these occasions my peril made me acutely aware of the aggressive hostility of the environment, and of my solitary condition. In these moods, books were a great solace, particularly books written by men who had survived, mainly by force of will, conditions every bit as desperate as mine, or worse.

In the beginning of my underground life, I ate two or three meals a day; but very soon, one sufficed. And I ate that meal only when I was hungry. My alimentary rhythm was quickly modified; what I considered my breakfast became in reality my lunch and dinner as well, for I usually went to bed very soon afterwards. Soon eating, though an important event in my day, became not a pleasant diversion, but a disagreeable duty. I noticed that my strength was failing, that I was losing weight, and that my diet was unbalanced, lacking certain essential vitamins. So I forced myself to eat—in order to survive.

When I felt weak and depressed I realized that I needed a tonic. When my back ached—the base of the spine pained me dreadfully towards the end of the experiment, caused no doubt by the more or less sedentary life I led—I thought of aspirin and how it could relieve that sometimes frighteningly acute pain. (Frightening, because it suggested paralysis, and I realized that, paralyzed, there would be no getting me through the narrow and twisting cat hole.) But I abstained from taking any kind of medicine. I had laid down the rule that I should take no medicine during my long night because I did not want to modify in any way the biological conditions of the experiment. For this reason I had taken no medicine down with me, except for a small first-aid kit, which remained untouched. For the same reason I had forbidden myself any tonic or vitamin additive when making up my provisions.

My major problem turned out to be my footgear. I had brought down four pairs of lined "house-shoes" for indoor wear, these having synthetic foam-rubber soles and waterproofed canvas bodies lined with down. For outside wear, the manufacturer had recommended a kind of outer shoe to wear over these, recalling old-fashioned spats, to which stout leather soles had been affixed. But from the very first days I discovered that my footgear would not possibly protect me against the thin sheet of water that covered the floor of my tent. The result was that during my entire stay underground I existed somehow with damp feet at best, and towards the end more than damp, soaked in icy water.

And the 9m water in the tent constantly increased in volume. The floor had a central seam, through which water oozed whenever I stepped on it. I wore two pairs of woolen socks; but of what use were they since they were always soaking wet? Having the wrong footwear might well have caused my death. And besides the water that penetrated from the outside, there was the humidity caused by perspiration—which, as I had learned in their books, was one of the chief clothing problems of Arctic explorers.

Wet feet no doubt contributed to the lowering of my body temperature. In the beginning I regularly took my temperature, which I wanted to record and compare with the graph of my heartbeat. But try as I would, the mercury in those thermometers would not rise above 97°F. I decided that my thermometers were defective, or were the wrong kind for the surrounding atmosphere, always hovering close to the freezing point. It was useless in any case to try warming them over my camp stove or inside the sleeping bag. So I decided not to pay any attention to what they recorded. When examined at the end of the experiment, the thermometers were found to be quite accurate. My skin temperature had actually sunk to 97°F. I was in a condition of semi-hibernation, what the doctors call hypothermia.

I lived in my subterranean retreat rather like a groundhog in winter, with lowered temperature, slowed-down movements, metabolism half dormant, auditory and visual faculties diminished.

I never suffered from claustrophobia, but I was subject to dizziness towards the end of my experiment. Sometimes when I went out on the moraine for supplies I would suddenly lose my balance, and twice barely saved myself from a fall that could have been fatal. As these spells of dizziness became more frequent, I went out on the moraine only when absolutely necessary. My universe shrank, and by the time my experiment "beyond time" had ended and my friends came down to fetch me, it was comprised exclusively of the space inside my tent.

Yes, my tent became my universe. Its effect upon my mind was remarkable. When I left the light bulb on and went outside, the tent glowed in the cold darkness with a redness that was singularly comforting. From the moraine I often looked back at it with a feeling of love. It represented security and shelter —no matter how specious that security and shelter, which was threatened constantly by the cave-ins of rock and ice. But it was my hearth and home and I loved it accordingly, feeling that thanks to it I could hold out against the hostile elements surrounding it. The occasionally terrifying sensation of infinite space that the impenetrable darkness of the cavern gave me vanished when I was inside my tent, even though the stars did not turn overhead and the days and nights did not succeed each other as they do over all the other tents in the world. My tent was outside the world. It was an entity in itself.

And the night never came to an end, but was always there, silent and eternal. The subterranean night is different from night on the earth's surface, for it is absolute, whereas on the surface, no matter how dark it is, there is always a glimmer of twilight on the horizon, or of stars in the firmament. In the cave, nothing is visible. In this dark void I sometimes felt disembodied, as if nothing subsisted but my mind, my thoughts. There were times when my mind reeled and I felt close to insanity, but very quickly I recovered self-control.

Even at the worst moments I never forgot my place in the scheme of things. There I was, a little man in a vast cavern camped on a subterranean glacier, alone in an environment that seemed inert. Yet I, as a geologist, was well aware that this matter had its own dynamics. It existed, had existed, and would exist. I was well aware that in the part of the world where I was, the oceans had been and had left sediments which produced the mountain ranges; life reigned in those ocean depths, then became extinguished when the continents appeared. I also knew that these mountains would in their turn disappear and make room for other oceans where life would be reborn in forms still more evolved. It would take millions of years; these changes in nature could not be perceptible on the scale of man but rather would be of another order. Our lives are too brief even to perceive that other forms of life are in evolution. For man, the world remains unchanged. Only astronomy and geology provide us with our dimension and set us properly in time and space. All nature is in a state of becoming. Yet here in the cave it seemed to be immobile, as if spellbound for eternity.

THE WORST JOURNEY IN THE WORLD
by Apsley Cherry-Garrard

The title may sound presumptuous—until you actually read Apsley Cherry-Garrard's immortal account of his Antarctic exploration with Scott between 1910 and 1913. It is hard to imagine more terrifying physical trials than those endured by the heroes of this expedition, and in Cherry-Garrard they found a chronicler who shared the stoic qualities of his colleagues and coupled them with an intensely graphic narrative gift. The extracts that follow are taken from "The

Winter Journey" which Cherry-Garrard made in June 1911, accompanied by Dr. Edward (Bill) Wilson and Henry (Birdie) Bowers in pursuit of the breeding grounds of the Emperor Penguin. Both Wilson and Bowers were to die, along with Scott, on their return from the South Pole nine months later.

~~~~~~~~~~~~~~~~~~~~~~~~~~~~~~~~~~~~~

Three men, one of whom at any rate is feeling a little frightened, stand panting and sweating out in McMurdo Sound. They have two sledges, one tied behind the other, and these sledges are piled high with sleeping bags and camping equipment, six weeks' provisions, and a venesta case full of scientific gear for pickling and preserving. In addition there is a pickaxe, ice axes, an Alpine rope, a large piece of green Willesden canvas and a bit of board. Our weights for such traveling are enormous—253 lbs. a man. It is midday but it is pitchy dark, and it is not warm.

What is this venture? Why is the embryo of the Emperor Penguin so important to Science? And why should three sane and common-sense explorers be sledging away on a winter's night to a Cape which has only been visited before in daylight, and then with very great difficulty?

The knowledge the world possessed at this time of the Emperor Penguin was mainly due to Wilson. But it is because the Emperor is probably the most primitive bird in existence that the working out of his embryology is so important. The embryo of an Emperor may prove the missing link between birds and the reptiles from which birds have sprung. Only one rookery of Emperor Penguins had been found at this date, and this was on the sea ice inside a little bay of the Barrier edge at Cape Crozier, which was guarded by miles of some of the biggest pressure in the Antarctic. Chicks had been found in September, so Wilson reckoned that the eggs must have been laid in the beginning of July.

And so we started just after midwinter—the weirdest bird's-nesting expedition that has ever been or ever will be.

The horror of the nineteen days it took us to travel from Cape Evans to Cape Crozier would have to be re-experienced to be appreciated; and anyone would be a fool who went again: it is not possible to describe it. The weeks which followed them were comparative bliss, not because later our conditions were better—they were far worse—but because we were callous. I for one had come to that point of suffering at which I did not really care if only I could die without much pain. They talk of the heroism of the dying—they little know—it would be so easy to die, a dose of morphia, a friendly crevasse, and blissful sleep. The trouble is to go on . . .

It was the darkness that did it. I don't believe minus seventy temperatures would be bad in daylight, not comparatively bad, when you could see where you were going, where you were stepping, where the sledge straps were, the cooker, the primus, the food; could see your footsteps lately trodden deep into the soft snow that you might find your way back to the rest of your load; could see the lashings of the food bags; could read a compass without striking three or four different boxes to find one dry match; could read your watch to see if the blissful moment of getting out of your bag was come without groping in the snow all about; when it would not take you five minutes to lash up the door of the tent, and five hours to get started in the morning.

But in these days we were never less than four hours from the moment when Bill cried "Time to get up" to the time when we got into our harness. It took two men to get one man into his harness, and was all they could do, for the canvas was frozen and our clothes were frozen until sometimes not even two men could bend them into the required shape.

The trouble is sweat and breath. I never knew before how much of the body's waste comes out through the pores of the skin. On the most bitter days, when we had to camp before we had done a four-hour march in order to nurse back our frozen feet, it seemed that we must be sweating. And all this sweat, instead of passing away through the porous wool of our clothing and gradually drying off us, froze and accumulated. It passed just away from our flesh and then became ice: we shook plenty of snow and ice down from inside our trousers every time we changed our footgear, and we could have shaken it from our vests and from between our vests and shirts, but of course we could not strip to this extent. But when we got into our sleeping bags, if we were fortunate, we became warm enough during the night to thaw this ice; part remained in our clothes, part passed into the skins of our sleeping bags, and soon both were sheets of armor plate.

As for our breath—in the daytime it did nothing worse than cover the lower parts of our faces with ice and solder our balaclavas tightly to our heads. It was no good trying to get your balaclava off until you had had the primus going quite a long time, and then you could throw your breath about if you wished. The trouble really began in your sleeping bag, for it was far too cold to keep a hole open through which to breathe. So all night long our breath froze into the skins, and our respiration became quicker and quicker as the air in our bags got fouler and fouler: it was never possible to make a match strike or burn inside our bags!

Of course we were not iced up all at once: it took several days of this kind of thing before we really got into big difficulties on this score. It was not until I got out of the tent one morning fully ready to pack the sledge that I realized the possibilities ahead. We had had our breakfast, struggled into our footgear, and squared up inside the tent, which was comparatively warm. Once outside, I raised my head to look around and found I could not move it back. My clothing had frozen hard as I stood—perhaps fifteen seconds. For four hours I had to pull with my head stuck up, and from that time we all took care to bend down into a pulling position before being frozen in.

When we tried to start on June 30th we found we could not move both sledges together. There was nothing for it but to take one on at a time and come back for the other. This has often been done in daylight when the only risks run are those of blizzards which may spring up suddenly and obliterate tracks.

Now in darkness it was more complicated. From 11 a.m. to 3 p.m. there was enough light to see the big holes made by our feet, and we took on one sledge, trudged back in our tracks, and brought on the second. Of course in this relay work we covered three miles in distance for every one mile forward, and even the single sledges were very hard pulling. When we lunched the temperature was −61 degrees. After lunch the little light had gone, and we carried a naked lighted candle back with us when we went to find our second sledge. It was the weirdest kind of procession, three frozen men and a little pool of light. Generally we steered by Jupiter, and I never see him now without recalling his friendship in those days.

We were very silent, it was not very easy to talk: but sledging is always a silent business. Do things slowly, always slowly, that was the burden of Wilson's leadership: and every now and then the question, Shall we go on? and the answer Yes. "I think we are all right as long as our appetites are good," said Bill. Always patient, self-possessed, unruffled, he was the only man on earth, I believe, who could have led this journey.

In civilization men are taken at their own valuation because there are so many ways of concealment, and there is so little time, perhaps even so little understanding. Not so down south. These two men went through the Winter Journey and lived; later they went through the Polar Journey and died. They were gold, pure, shining, unalloyed. Words cannot express how good their companionship was.

Through all these days, and those which were to follow—the worst, I suppose, in their dark severity that men have ever come through alive—no single hasty or angry word passed their lips. When, later, we were sure, so far as we can be sure of anything, that we must die, they were cheerful, and so far as I can judge their songs and cheery words were quite unforced. Nor were they ever flurried, though always as quick as the conditions would allow in moments of emergency. It is hard that often such men must go first when others far less worthy remain.

The temperature on the night of July 6th was −75.8 degrees, and I will not pretend that it did not convince me that Dante was right when he placed the circles of ice below the circles of fire. Still we slept sometimes, and always we lay for seven hours. Again and again Bill asked us how about going back, and always we said no. Yet there was nothing I should have liked better: I was quite sure that to dream of Cape Crozier was the wildest lunacy. That day we had advanced 1 1/2 miles by the utmost labor, and the usual relay work. This was quite a good march—and Cape Crozier is 67 miles from Cape Evans!

More than once in my short life have I been struck by the value of the man who is blind to what appears to be a common-sense certainty; he achieves the impossible. We never spoke our thoughts; we discussed the Age of Stone which was to come, when we built our cozy warm rock hut on the slopes of Mount Terror, and ran our stove with penguin blubber, and pickled little Emperors in warmth and dryness. We were quite intelligent people, and we must all have known that we were not going to see the penguins and that it was folly to go forward. And yet with quiet perseverance, in perfect friendship, almost with gentleness those two men led on. I just did what I was told.

It is desirable that the body should work, feed and sleep at regular hours, and this is too often forgotten when sledging. But just now we found we were unable to fit 8 hours' marching and 7 hours in our sleeping bags into a 24-hour day: the routine camp work took more than 9 hours, such were the conditions. We therefore ceased to observe the quite imaginary difference between night and day, and it was noon on Friday (July 7th) before we got away. The temperature was −68 degrees and there was a thick white fog; we camped at 10 P.M. after managing 1 3/4 miles for the day. But what a relief. Instead of laboring away, our hearts were beating more naturally; it was easier to camp, we had some feeling in our hands, and our feet had not gone to sleep. Birdie swung the thermometer and found it only −55 degrees. "Now if we tell people that to get only eighty-seven degrees of frost can be an enormous relief, they simply won't believe us," I remember saying. Perhaps you won't, but it was, all the same; and I wrote that night: "There is something, after all, rather good in doing something never done before."

Later, after further ordeals, the three explorers succeeded in reaching Cape Crozier and collecting the precious penguin eggs. They built an igloo to protect themselves from the elements. And then came the supreme test of their fortitude . . .

All day it had been blowing a nasty cold wind with a temperature between −20 and −30 degrees, which we felt a good deal. Now it began to get worse. The weather was getting thick, and things did not look very nice when we started up to find our tent. Soon it was blowing Force 4, and soon we missed our way entirely. We got right up above the patch of rocks which marked our igloo and only found it after a good deal of search.

I have heard tell of an English officer at the Dardanelles who was left, blinded, in no man's land between the English and Turkish trenches. Moving only at night, and having no sense to tell him which were his own trenches, he was fired at by Turk and English alike as he groped his ghastly way to and from them. Thus he spent days and nights until, one night, he crawled towards the English trenches, to be fired at as usual. "Oh God! what can I do!" someone heard him say, and he was brought in.

Such extremity of suffering cannot be measured; madness or death may give relief. But this I know: we on this journey were already beginning to think of death as a friend. As we groped our way back that night, sleepless, icy, and dog-tired in the dark and the wind and the drift, a crevasse seemed almost a friendly gift.

"Things must improve," said Bill the next day. After all, there was much for which to be thankful. I don't think anybody could have made a better igloo with the hard snow blocks and rocks which were all we had; we would get it airtight by degrees. The blubber stove was working, and we had fuel for it. We had also found a way down to the penguins and had three complete, though frozen, eggs; two others, which had been in my mitts, smashed when I fell about because I could not wear spectacles. Also, the twilight given by the sun below the horizon at noon was getting longer. We felt no particular uneasiness. Our tent was well dug in, and was also held down by rocks and by the heavy tank off the sledge which were placed on the skirting as additional security. We felt that no power on earth could move the thick walls of our igloo, nor drag the canvas roof from the middle of the embankment into which it was packed and lashed.

I do not know what time it was when I woke up. It was calm, with that absolute silence which can be so soothing or so terrible as circumstances dictate. Then there came a sob of wind, and all was still again. Ten minutes, and it was blowing as though the world was having a fit of hysterics. The earth was torn in pieces; the indescribable fury and roar of it all cannot be imagined.

"Bill, Bill, the tent has gone," was the next I remember—from Bowers shouting at us again and again through the door. It is always these early morning shocks which hit one hardest: our slow minds suggested that this might mean a particularly lingering form of death. Journey after journey Birdie and I fought our way across the few yards which had separated the tent from the igloo door. I have never understood why so much of our gear which was in the tent remained, even in the lee of the igloo. The place where the tent had been was littered with gear, and when we came to reckon up afterward we had everything except the bottom piece of the cooker, and the top of the outer cooker. We never saw these again. The most wonderful thing of all was that our finnesko were lying where they were left, which happened to be on the ground in the part of the tent which was under the lee of the igloo. Also Birdie's bag of personal gear was there, and a tin of sweets.

To get that gear in, we fought against solid walls of black snow which flowed past us and tried to hurl us down the slope. Once started, nothing could have stopped us. I saw Birdie knocked over once, but he clawed his way back just in time. Having passed everything we could find in to Bill, we got back into the igloo, and started to collect things together, including our very disheveled minds.

There was no doubt that we were in the devil of a mess, and it was not altogether our fault. We had had to put our igloo more or less where we could get rocks with which to build it. Very naturally we had given both our tent and igloo all the shelter we could from the full force of the wind, and now it seemed we were in danger not because they were in the wind, but because they were not sufficiently in it. The main force of the hurricane, deflected by the ridge behind, fled over our heads and appeared to form, by suction, a vacuum below. Our tent had either been sucked upward into this, or had been blown away because some of it was in the wind while some of it was not. The roof of our igloo was being wrenched upward and then dropped back with great crashes: the drift was spouting in—not, it seemed, because it was blown in from outside, but because it was sucked in from within: the lee, not the weather, wall was the worst. Already everything was six or eight inches under snow.

Very soon we began to be alarmed about the igloo. For some time the heavy snow blocks we had heaved up onto the canvas roof kept it weighted down. But it seemed that they were being gradually moved off by the hurricane. The tension became well-nigh unendurable; the waiting in all that welter of noise was maddening. Minute after minute, hour after hour—those snow blocks were off now anyway, and the roof was smashed up and down—no canvas ever made could stand it indefinitely.

We got a meal that Saturday morning—our last for a very long time, as it happened. Oil being of such importance to us, we tried to use the blubber stove, but after several preliminary spasms it came to pieces in our hands, some solder having melted; and a very good thing too, I thought, for it was more dangerous than useful. We finished cooking our meal on the primus. Two bits of the cooker having been blown away, we had to balance it on the primus as best we could. We then settled that in view of the shortage of oil, we would not have another meal for as long as possible. As a matter of fact, God settled that for us.

We did all we could to stop up the places where the drift was coming in, plugging the holes with our socks, mitts and other clothing. But it was no real good. Our igloo was a vacuum which was filling itself up as soon as possible; and when snow was not coming in, a fine black moraine dust took its place, covering us and everything. For twenty-four hours we waited for the roof to go; things were so bad now that we dared not unlash the door.

Many hours before, Bill had told us that if the roof went, he considered that our best chance would be to roll over in our sleeping bags until we were lying on the openings, and get frozen and drifted in.

Gradually the situation got more desperate. The distance between the taut-sucked canvas and the sledge on which it should have been resting became greater, and this must have been due to the stretching of the canvas itself and the loss of the snow blocks on the top: it was not drawing out of the walls. The crashes as it dropped and banged out again were louder. There was more snow coming through the walls, though all our loose mitts, socks and smaller clothing were stuffed into the worst places: our pajama jackets were stuffed between the roof and the rocks over the door. The rocks were lifting and shaking here till we thought they would fall.

And then it went.

Birdie was over by the door, where the canvas which was bent over the lintel board was working worse than anywhere else. Bill was practically out of his bag pressing against some part with a long stick of some kind. I don't know what I was doing but I was half out of and half in my bag.

The top of the door opened in little slits and that green Willesden canvas flapped into hundreds of little fragments in fewer seconds than it takes to read this. The uproar of it all was indescribable. Even above the savage thunder of that great wind on the mountain came the lash of the canvas as it was whipped to tiny little strips. The highest rocks which we had built into our walls fell upon us, and a sheet of drift came in.

Birdie dived for his sleeping bag and eventually got in, together with a terrible lot of drift. Bill also, but he was better off; I was already half into mine and all right, so I turned to help Bill. "Get into your own," he shouted, and when I continued to try and help him, he leaned over until his mouth was against my ear. *"Please*, Cherry," he said, and his voice was terribly anxious. I know he felt responsible—feared it was he who had brought us to this ghastly end.

The next I knew was Bowers' head across Bill's body. "We're all right," he yelled, and we answered in the affirmative. Despite the fact that we knew we only said so because we knew we were all wrong, this statement was helpful. Then we turned our bags over as far as possible, so that the bottom of the bag was uppermost and the flaps were more or less beneath us. And we lay and thought, and sometimes we sang.

I can well believe that neither of my companions gave up hope for an instant. They must have been frightened, but they were never disturbed. As for me, I never had any hope at all; and when the roof went I felt that this was the end. What else could I think? We had spent days in reaching this place through the darkness in cold such as had never been experienced by human beings. We had been out for four weeks under conditions in which no man had existed previously for more than a few days, if that. During this time we had seldom slept except from sheer physical exhaustion, as men sleep on the rack; and every minute of it we had been fighting for the bedrock necessaries of bare existence, and always in the dark. We had kept ourselves going by enormous care of our feet and hands and bodies, by burning oil, and by having plenty of hot fatty food. Now we had no tent, one tin of oil left out of six, and only part of our cooker. When we were lucky and not too cold we could almost wring water from our clothes, and directly we got out of our sleeping bags we were frozen into solid sheets of armored ice. In cold temperatures with all the advantages of a tent over our heads we were already taking more than an hour of fierce struggling and cramp to get into our sleeping bags—so frozen were they and so long did it take us to thaw our way in. No! Without the tent we were dead men.

And there seemed not one chance in a million that we would ever see our tent again. We were 900 feet up on the mountainside, and the wind blew about as hard as a wind can blow straight out to sea. First there was a steep slope, so hard that a pick made little impression upon it, so slippery that if you started down in finnesko you never could stop. This ended in a great ice cliff some hundreds of feet high, and then came miles of pressure ridges, crevassed and tumbled, in which you might as well look for a daisy as a tent—and after that the open sea. The chances, however, were that the tent had just been taken up into the air and dropped somewhere in this sea well on the way to New Zealand. Obviously the tent was gone.

Face to face with real death one does not think of the things that torment the bad people in the tracts and fill the good people with bliss. I might have speculated on my chances of going to Heaven; but candidly, I did not care. I could not have wept if I had tried. I had no wish to review the evils of my past. But the past did seem to have been a bit wasted. The road to Hell may be paved with good intentions; the road to Heaven is paved with lost opportunities.

I wanted those years over again. What fun I would have with them, what glorious fun! It was a pity. Well has the Persian said that when we come to die we, remembering that God is merciful, will gnaw our elbows with remorse for thinking of the things we have not done for fear of the Day of Judgment.

And I wanted peaches and syrup—badly. We had them at the hut, sweeter and more luscious than you can imagine. And we had been without sugar for a month. Yes—especially the syrup.

Thus impiously I set out to die, making up my mind that I was not going to try and keep warm, that it might not take too long, and thinking I would try and get some morphia from the medical case if it got very bad. Not a bit heroic, and entirely true! Yes, comfortable, warm reader! Men do not fear death; they fear the pain of dying.

In Praise of Insomnia

Here are two tributes to the often unrecognized pleasures of a sleepless night. The first is from Travels with a Donkey in the Cevennes *by Robert Louis Stevenson, published in 1879, and the second is an essay which Brian Aldiss wrote in 1972. Although a century separates Stevenson's "I have not often enjoyed a more serene possession of myself, nor felt more independent of material aids" and Aldiss' "It is at night . . . that the mind is most clear, that we are most able to hold all our life in the palm of our skull," the mood and the viewpoint are identical.*

A NIGHT AMONG THE PINES
by Robert Louis Stevenson

Night is a dead monotonous period under a roof; but in the open world it passes lightly, with its stars and dews and perfumes, and the hours are marked by changes in the fact of Nature. What seems a kind of temporal death to people choked between walls and curtains is only a light and living slumber to the man who sleeps afield. All night long he can hear Nature breathing deeply and freely; even as she takes her rest, she turns and smiles; and there is one stirring hour unknown to those who dwell in houses, when a wakeful influence goes abroad over the sleeping hemisphere, and all the outdoor world are on their feet. It is then that the cock first crows, not this time to announce the dawn, but like a cheerful watchman speeding the course of night. Cattle awake on the meadows; sheep break their fast on dewy hillsides, and change to a new lair among the ferns; and houseless men, who have lain down with the fowls, open their dim eyes and behold the beauty of the night.

At what inaudible summons, at what gentle touch of Nature, are all these sleepers thus recalled in the same hour to life? Do the stars rain down an influence, or do we share some thrill of mother earth below our resting bodies? Even shepherds and old country-folk, who are the deepest read in these arcana, have not a guess as to the means or purpose of this nightly resurrection. Towards two in the morning they declare the thing takes place; and neither know nor inquire further. And at least it is a pleasant incident. We are disturbed in our slumber only, like the luxurious Montaigne, "that we may the better and more sensibly relish it." We have a moment to look upon the stars. And there is a special pleasure for some minds in the reflection that we share the impulse with all outdoor creatures in our neighbourhood, that we have escaped out of the Bastille of civilisation, and are become, for the time being, a mere kindly animal and a sheep of Nature's flock.

When that hour came to me among the pines, I wakened thirsty. My tin was standing by me half full of water. I emptied it at a draught; and feeling broad awake after this internal cold aspersion, sat upright to make a cigarette. The stars were clear, coloured, and jewel-like, but not frosty. A faint silvery vapour stood for the Milky Way. All around me the black fir-points stood upright and stock-still. By the whiteness of the pack-saddle, I could see Modestine walking round and round at the length of her tether; I could hear her steadily munching at the sward; but there was not another sound, save the indescribable quiet talk of the runnel over the stones. I lay lazily smoking and studying the colour of the sky, as we call the void of space, from where it showed a reddish grey behind the pines to where it showed a glossy blue-black between the stars. As if to be more like a pedlar, I wear a silver ring. This I could see faintly shining as I raised or lowered the cigarette; and at each whiff the inside of my hand was illuminated, and became for a second the highest light in the landscape.

A faint wind, more like a moving coolness than a stream of air, passed down the glade from time to time; so that even in my great chamber the air was being renewed all night long. I thought with horror of the inn at Chasserades and the congregated nightcaps; with horror of the nocturnal prowesses of clerks and students; of hot theatres and pass-keys and close rooms. I have not often enjoyed a more serene possession of myself, nor felt more independent of material aids. The outer world, from which we cower into our houses, seemed after all a gentle habitable place; and night after night a man's bed, it seemed, was laid and waiting for him in the fields, where God keeps an open house. I thought I had rediscovered one of those truths which are revealed to savages and hid from political economists: at the least, I had discovered a new pleasure for myself. And yet even while I was exulting in my solitude I became aware of a strange lack. I wished a companion to lie near me in the starlight, silent and not moving, but ever within touch. For there is a fellowship more quiet even than solitude, and which, rightly understood, is solitude made perfect. And to live out of doors with the woman a man loves is of all lives the most complete and free.

As I thus lay, between content and longing, a faint noise stole towards me through the pines. I thought, at first, it was the crowing of cocks or the barking of dogs at some very distant farm; but steadily and gradually it took articulate shape in my ears, until I became aware that a passenger was going by upon the high-road in the valley, and singing loudly as he went. There was more of good-will than grace in his performance; but he trolled with ample lungs; and the sound of his voice took hold upon the hillside and set the air shaking in the leafy glens. I have heard people passing by night in sleeping cities; some of them sang; one, I remember, played loudly on the bagpipes. I have heard the rattle of a cart or carriage spring up suddenly after hours of stillness, and pass, for some minutes, within the range of my hearing as I lay abed. There is a romance about all who are abroad in the black hours, and with something of a thrill we try to guess their business. But here the romance was double: first, this glad passenger, lit internally with wine, who sent up his voice in music through the night; and then I, on the other hand, buckled into my sack, and smoking alone in the pine-woods between four and five thousand feet towards the stars.

When I awoke again, many of the stars had disappeared; only the stronger companions of the night still burned visibly over-head; and away towards the east I saw a faint haze of light upon the horizon, such as had been the Milky Way when I was last awake. Day was at hand. I lit my lantern, and by its glow-worm light put on my boots and gaiters; then I broke up some bread for Modestine, filled my can at the water-tap, and lit my spirit-lamp to boil myself some chocolate. The blue darkness lay long in the glade where I had so sweetly slumbered; and soon there was a broad streak of orange melting into gold along the mountain-tops of Vivarais. A solemn glee possessed my mind at this gradual and lovely coming in of day.

REFLECTIONS OF AN ARDENT INSOMNIAC
by Brian Aldiss

Memory is the poor man's art. As an ardent insomniac, I was wide awake the other morning at five o'clock, and slipped out of the dark and silent house to take a walk down our avenue of beeches to the main road. Dawn was a newcomer in the sky, oozing through a slit in the cloud-cover like honey from a sandwich.

Suburbia has crept out to Southmoor. There is a new butcher's shop almost opposite the end of our drive. A light was burning in it, and had been all night, but it reminded me of the frisson I used to feel as a child in that hour before the dawn when human activity slowly gets going again.

There used to be a particular nervous pleasure at the sight of a butcher sprinkling sawdust over his floor, orange lights flicking on in bedroom windows, the first dog let on to the street. Later, there were gritty army dawns, with a mug of char coming up at six o'clock, when the guard changed; the first milkman clanking down the road, a man whistling to the sound of his own footsteps. These were all signs of that extraordinary event—more rather than less extraordinary by dint of its daily repetition—the revolution of Earth, bringing England back within reach of sun again.

Such grand sidereal events are more accessible at night. With humanity roosting, the processes of Earth come into their own. The air is fresh and still. A lone car, belting down the A420, is no more than a creaking cart—a pathetic little vehicle belonging to a species trying to make the best of its tenuous hold on the universe. There are lights along the road, but the brightest light is so feeble and transitory compared with the sun as to be laughable.

I was thinking of J. B. Priestley's new book, *Over the Long High Wall.* As he does, I regard myself as a time-haunted man. One does not have to accept his speculation that we are six-dimensional creatures to feel that we contain many sorts of time within us. He is surely right in holding that one of the worst evils of our century is our enslavement to clock-time, whereas all of us (unless we are mentally sick) acknowledge inwardly how free we are to move either back into that time which memory keeps or forward into that time which intellect keeps—the ability to live in the future is a very recent human skill.

Pleasure, more than ever before, is never at home, but headlong joy is ever on the wing.

It's at night, when perhaps we should be dreaming, that the mind is most clear, that we are most able to hold all our life in the palm of our skull. I don't know if anyone has ever pointed out that great attraction of insomnia before, but it is so; the night seems to release a little more of our vast backward inheritance of instincts and feelings. Perhaps, as with the dawn, a little honey is allowed to ooze between the lips of the sandwich, a little of the stuff of dreams to drip into the waking mind.

Anyhow, as I was walking back up the drive, I was composing an essay, rather in the Hazlitt manner. In Praise of Human Consciousness. I am so appallingly naïve that merely *being aware* still surprises me as much as the diurnal revolution of the Earth. Who thought it all up, this whole amazing complexity of motion among which we move with such ease? Or, if No One thought it up, what a bit of luck for us that an Accident happened! Such a reflection recurs occasionally, mutatis mutandis, over the years. I remember it first struck me —and struck is the word I want—when I was about four or five, looking into our airing cupboard and seeing the clothes and bars of soap piled up in orderly fashion. Good Lord, thought I, or words to that effect, I suppose everything in the world must be to a purpose. But what purpose?

Well, if I am no nearer an answer now than I was then, at least I have never tired of the mystery.

A cock was crowing as I got back to the house—the last medieval sound in Southmoor. Freedom in the skull is always closely linked with precise coordination in orthodox space-time; even the longest and most momentous journeys start at some fiddling little time like 5:17. It was a secret Shakespeare knew: airy nothings must always have a local habitation and a name. My first glimpse of an eternal moment was through an airing cupboard door in East Dereham, Norfolk. Remembering makes us free of clock-time—but of course to be free forever from clock-time is to be disembodied, an airy nothing.

I wish I believed, as Priestley does, that consciousness continued after disembodiment or death, not forever, but for a long while. Three score years and ten is such a stingy ration of time, when there is so much time around. Perhaps that's why some of us are insomniacs; night is so precious that it would be pusillanimous to sleep all through it! A "bad night" is not always a bad thing.

ABOUT THE AUTHOR

HILARY RUBINSTEIN is a writer, editor and literary agent who lives in London with his wife and children. He is the only member of his family not to go into the Law, but that has not spared him the family's insomnia. In fact, the idea for this book came to him during one sleepless night and he says, "It's the only good idea I've ever had in the middle of the night."